HEARTFELT JOURNEY

A CARDIOLOGIST'S MEMOIRS

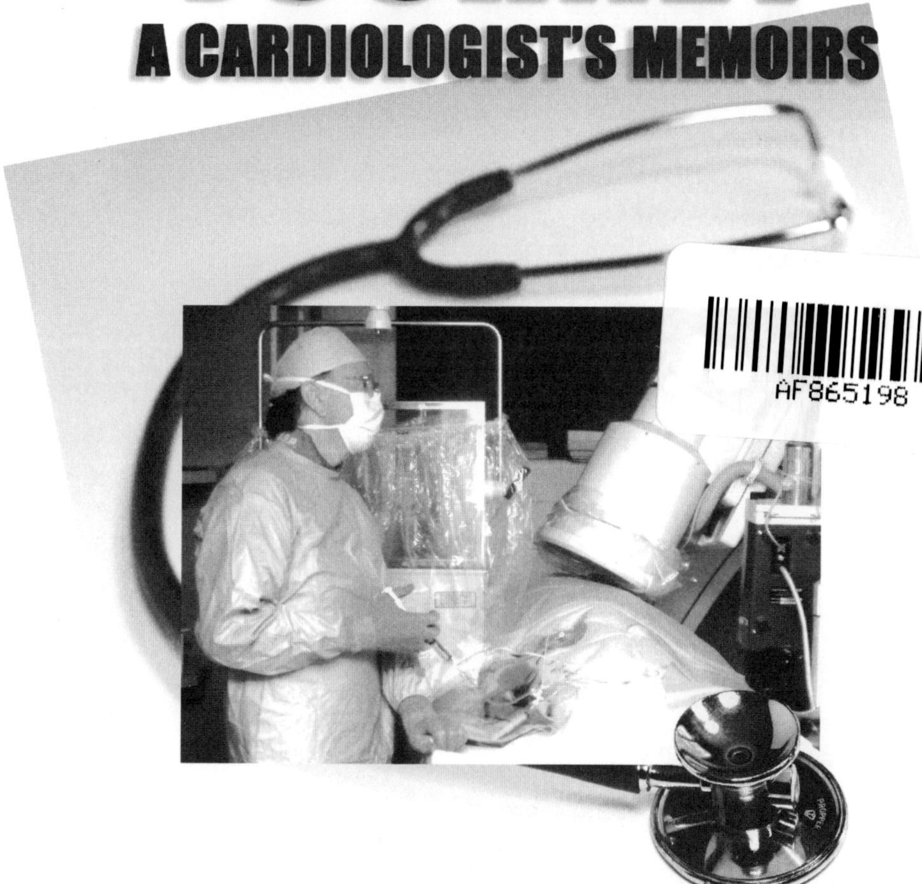

AF865198

LOWELL F. PETERSON, M.D.

Copyright© 2011 Peterson House

All rights reserved.
No part of this book may be
reproduced in any form without
permission of the author.

First Edition

ISBN Number: 0-9719128-5-4

Library of Congress Control Number:
2011906481

Published by:
PETERSON HOUSE
2627 Beechwood Court
Appleton, WI 54911
SRoseClear@aol.com

Book cover and interior design by
Camin Potts
GRAPHIC LIAISONS, LLC
Waupaca, WI 54981
cpottsdesign.com

Back cover photo by
James Gill
Wisconsin Public Television

Printed in the United States by
Worzalla Publishing Company
Stevens Point, WI 54481
www.worzalla.com

DEDICATION

My medical memoirs are dedicated with deep affection to my family—my wife, Mary; our children, Linda, James, Kristin, and Erik; our grandchildren, Kristin, Erin, and Ryan McKenzie, Hannah and Ella Peterson, Harry, Finn, and Mary O'Callaghan, Mayes, Elsa, and Beckett Peterson. They are my inspiration and my pride and joy.

Dedication iii

CONTENTS

Legacy—Historical Milestones in Cardiology ix

Author's Note xiii

Preface—An Incredible Journey xvii

Introduction xxi

Chapter One **BEGINNING THE JOURNEY** (1940-1954) 1

Chapter Two **LUTHER COLLEGE** (1954-1958) 9

Chapter Three **MEDICAL SCHOOL - THE FIRST DAY** (September 1958) 21

Chapter Four **THE EARLY DAYS** (1958) 25

Chapter Five **THE FIRST TWO YEARS** (1958-1959) 29

Chapter Six **THE CLINICAL YEARS** (1960-1962) 37

Chapter Seven **INTERNSHIP** (1962-1963) 49

Chapter Eight **AIR FORCE MEDICINE** (1963-1966) 59

Chapter Nine **INTERNAL MEDICINE RESIDENCY** (1966-1969) 71

Chapter Ten **CARDIOLOGY FELLOWSHIP** (1969-1970) 93

Chapter Eleven **THE APPLETON ADVENTURE BEGINS** (1970-1980) 105

Chapter Twelve **THE GLORY YEARS** (1980-1988) 119

Chapter Thirteen **THE OTHER SIDE OF THE STETHOSCOPE: ROLES REVERSE** (1988) 125

Chapter Fourteen **THE CULMINATION OF A LABOR OF LOVE** 137

VIGNETTES OF MEMORABLE PATIENTS 141

THE APPLETON HEART INSTITUTE—THE BIRTH OF A DREAM 155

ACKNOWLEDGMENTS 159

"To prevent disease,
to relieve suffering
and to heal the sick—
This is our work."
—Sir William Osler

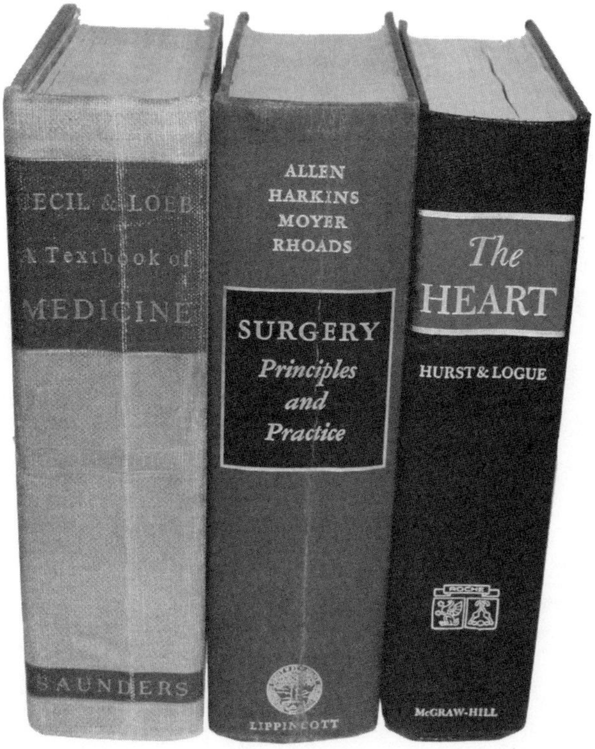

"To cure sometimes,
to relieve often,
to comfort always."
—Anonymous

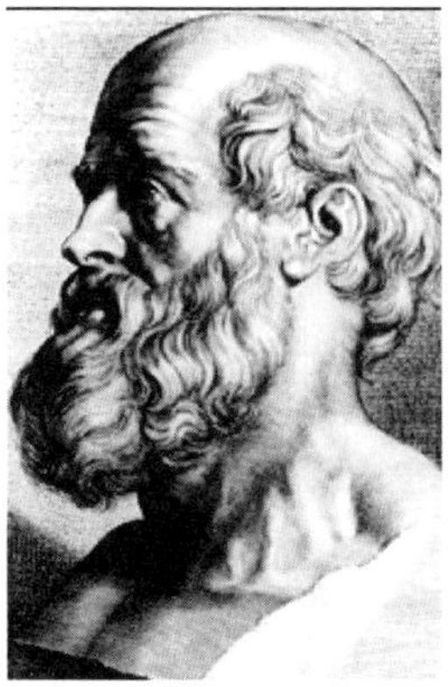

Hippocrates

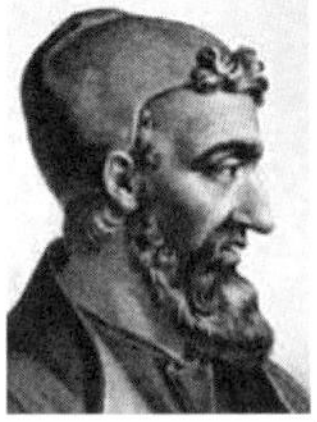

Galen

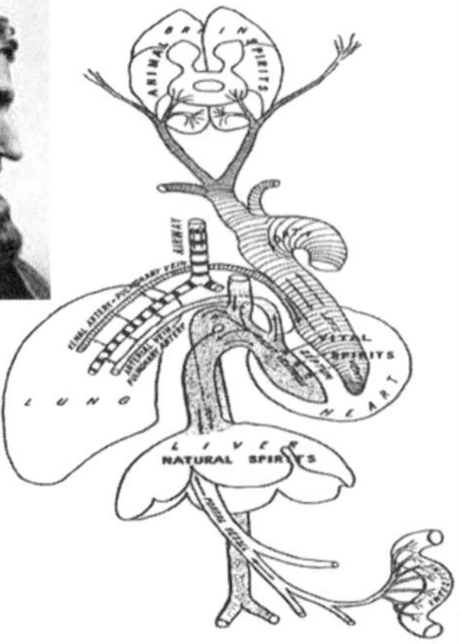

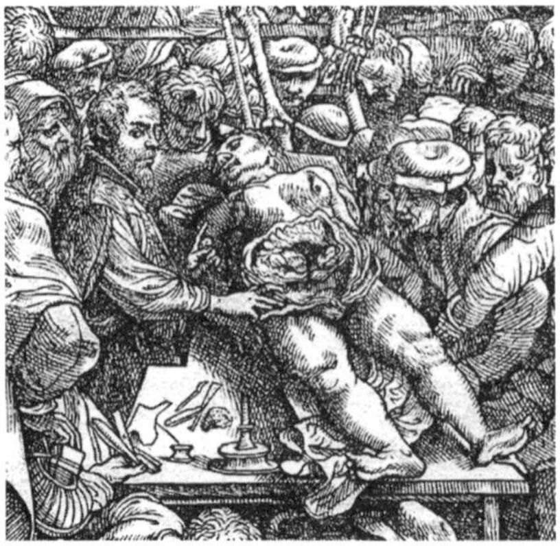

Andreas Vesalius

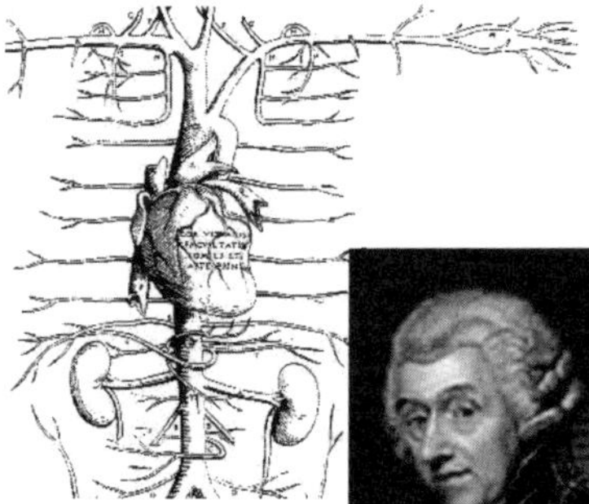

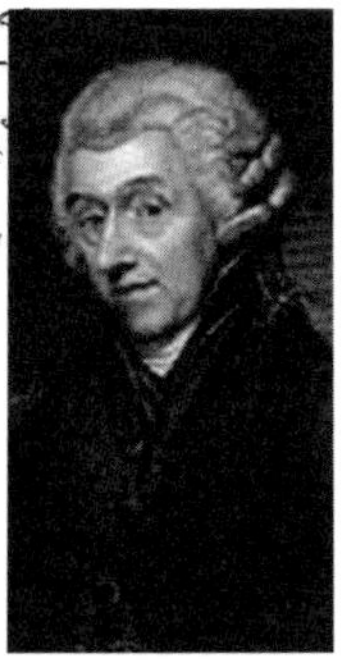

William Heberden

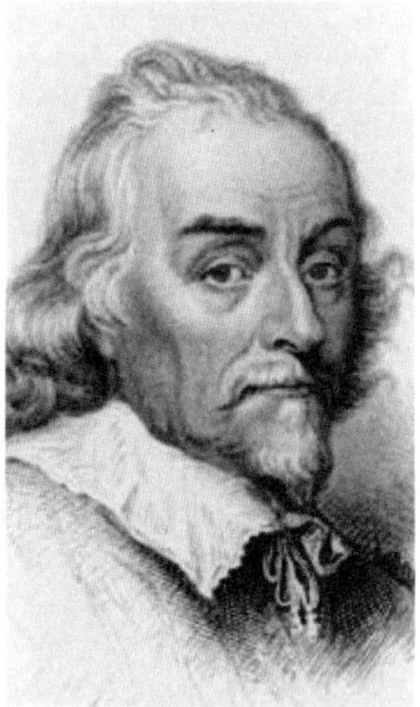

William Harvey

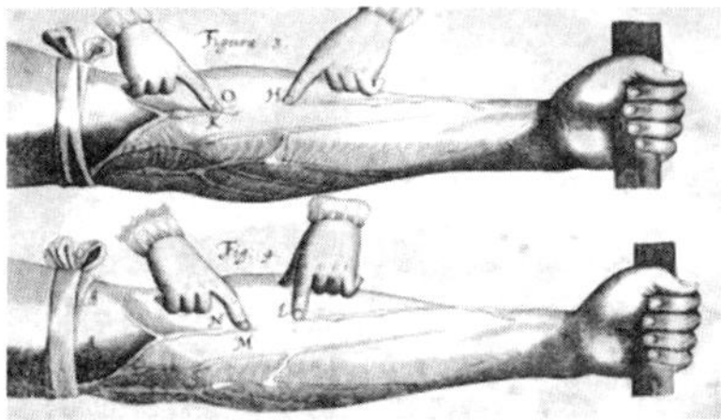

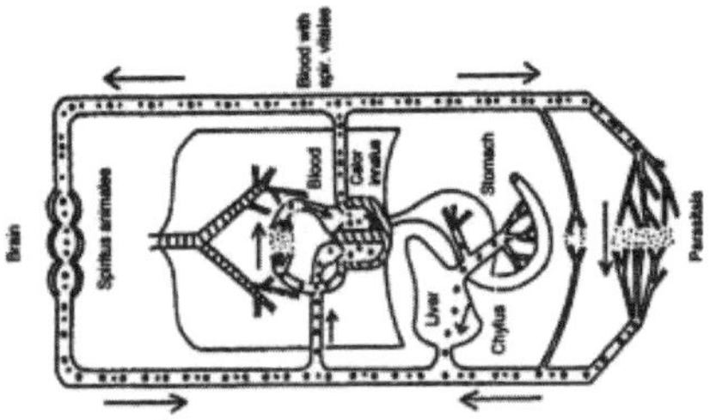

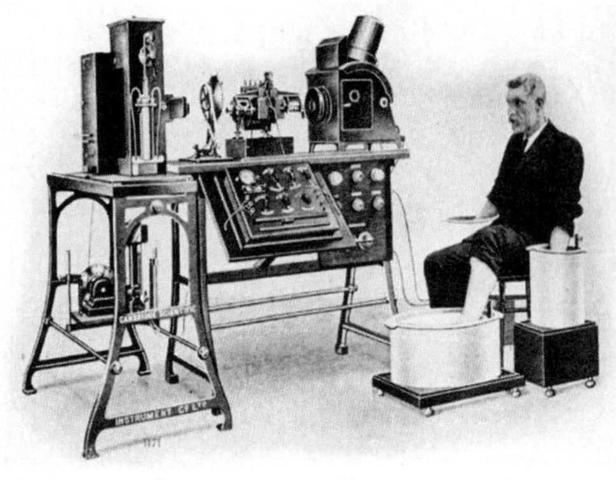

Einthoven's first electrocardiogram machine

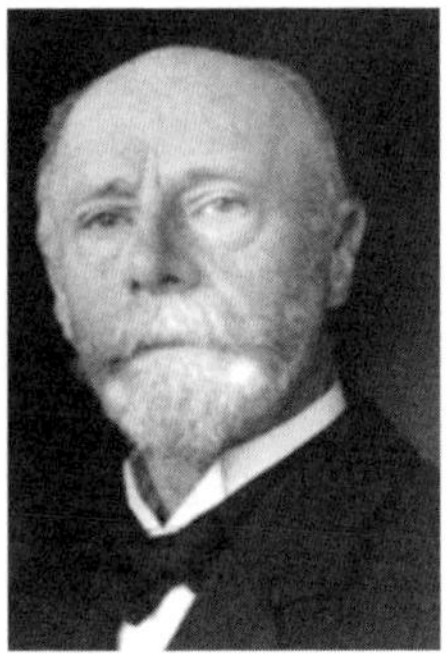

Einthoven

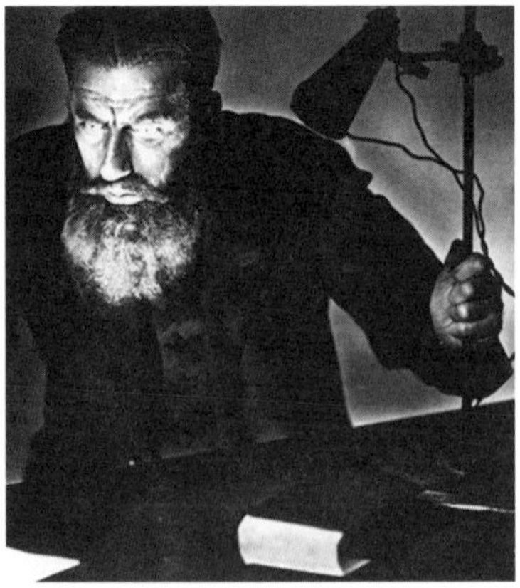

Wilhelm Roentgen

LEGACY

HISTORICAL MILESTONES IN CARDIOLOGY

"Life is short and the art is long; the occasion fleeting; experience fallacious; and judgement difficult."

—Hippocrates

Hippocrates, the Father of Medicine (460-377 B.C.) examined the heart by post-mortem dissection, but it would be more than 500 years before Galen (132-201 A.D.) described the anatomy and physiology of the heart. This remained the accepted dogma, imperfect as it was, until Andreas Vesalius (1514-1564) used comprehensive dissection to show that the arterial and venous systems were connected rather than separate circulations. William Harvey (1578-1657) used vivisection, the dissection of living animals, to describe the circulatory system and the coronary circulation.

William Heberden (1710-1801), describing a disease state of the heart in clinical terms for the first time, noted, *"There is a disorder of the breast marked with strong and peculiar symptoms, considerable for the kind of danger belonging to it, and not extremely rare. The sense of strangling, and the anxiety with which it is attended, may not improperly be called angina pectoris."*

The invention of the stethoscope in the 18th century, the sphygmomanometer in the 19th century, the discovery of X-ray by Roentgen in 1895, and the invention of the electrocardiogram in the early 1900s advanced the clinical evaluation of the cardiovascular system.

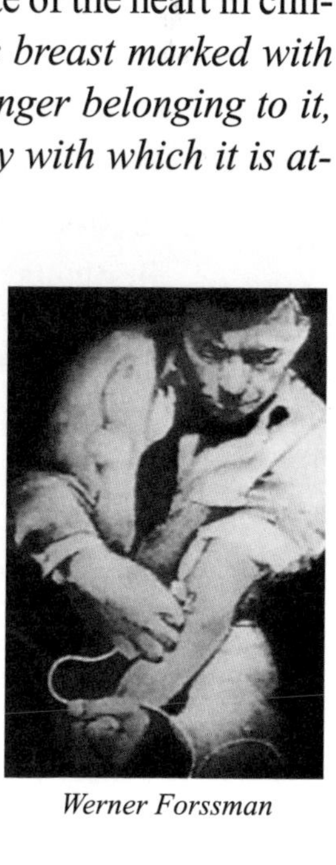
Werner Forssman

In 1929, Werner Forssman, in Germany, courageously passed a ureteral (urinary tract) catheter through a vein of his left arm and advanced the catheter invasively into his heart. He also showed the feasibility of injecting radiopaque chemicals via the catheter into the heart, recording these events by X-ray. Now, for the first time, it was possible to study the heart as a

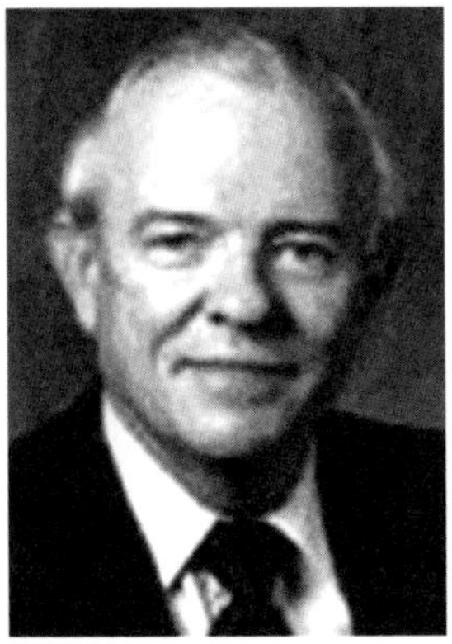

F. Mason Sones, Jr.

vital, functioning organ.

In 1958, Dr. Mason Sones discovered selective coronary artery arteriography, by accident, when a power injection of radiopaque contrast media in the central aorta suddenly whipped the catheter into the right coronary artery, outlining it in great detail (an anxiety provoking experience which he expected would lead to death of the patient—but, surprisingly, caused no adverse response). In 1962, Dr. Sones described the results of selective coronary arteriography in his first 1,000 cases. By 1996, 1,713,000 coronary catheterizations had been performed worldwide.

In the last 50 years of the 20th century an exponential number of contributions in the field of cardiology and cardiac surgery occurred, making it, not unreasonably, "The Golden Age of Cardiology". Of the countless advancements in this era, I have selected 15 examples of the major achievements:

1. Cardiac Catheterization and Coronary Arteriography
2. The Heart-Lung Pump Oxygenator (for circulatory and respiratory support during open-heart surgery)
3. Coronary Artery Bypass Grafting
4. External and Internal Cardiac Defibrillators (for life-threatening arrhythmias)
5. Percutaneous Transluminal Coronary Angioplasty (PTCA)
6. Echocardiography
7. Implantable Cardiac Pacemakers
8. Cardiac Transplantation
9. Thrombolytic Therapy of Acute Coronary Syndromes
10. Heart Valve and Aorto-Vascular Surgery Repair or Replacement
11. Coronary Stent Therapy of Acute and Chronic Coronary Syndromes
12. Arrhythmia Ablation Therapy
13. Nuclear Cardiac Function and Stress Test Imaging
14. Preventive Cardiac Interventional Therapy—Drugs, Diet, Lifestyle, Exercise
15. Sophisticated Drugs—Both Therapeutic and Preventive

AUTHOR'S NOTE

"A man cannot tell the whole truth about himself even if convinced that what he wrote would never be seen by others."

—Mark Twain
London Times, 23 May 1899

There was no sudden revelation or transfiguration, no blinding light on the road to Damascus, no voice emanating from a burning bush on a mountain that said it was my destiny to become a doctor. My path toward medicine was an evolutionary one, dependent on a combination of self-selecting personality traits and gut-wrenching decisions. In preparing to write this memoir—an idea of recording what I remembered while I still remembered it—it struck me that when I held a mirror up to my daily experiences in the trenches of the medical field, the reflections I saw were not of the fabled physician-as-healer, but more properly, a skilled and highly knowledgeable professional plying his trade. I suppose the sheer relentlessness of disease accounts for some of this disconnect. Day in and day out, a doctor confronts illness and does all he can to conquer it. While it's a noble task, it can be a tedious one. My experience as a doctor was never boring. It was by turns exhilarating, frustrating, horribly depressing, and miraculously profound—sometimes all in the span of 24 hours. But, as I trace my journey and catalogue my experiences, it occurs to me that the wonderful privilege I was given to help people while they were sick was never a pre-ordained "destiny".

How strange to find, then, as I jotted down every milestone on my road, I couldn't keep one thought from popping into my brain: "How amazing!" I was not in awe of myself, but I was awed by the fact that I had made this journey at all. At some point in life I imagine everyone looks around and wonders, "How did I get here?" Like many others who were also very fortunate in their choices, their opportunities, their family life, and their natural fortitude, it can be easy to view the successful results of many years' hard work as the natural endpoint: It's simply what was supposed to happen. But, don't believe it. Conscious decisions and the courage to carry those ideas to fruition were required in order to succeed.

In recording scenes of my professional life on paper, I don't aim to inspire future physicians or hope to swell hearts with gratitude for my noble profession (and, in turn for me). I simply want to record what happened and, at this late date, revel in the journey that I made. Hopefully, my experiences may cause others to reflect on their own pathways in life.

PREFACE

AN INCREDIBLE JOURNEY

I retired from the practice of medicine on February 1, 2009, 46 years and eight months after receiving my Doctor of Medicine degree—in May 1962—from the University of Wisconsin. I consider it a privilege to have served my fellowman in this profession, and I sincerely believe that I performed my mandated duties with intelligence, veracity, and compassion.

I was fortunate that my career spanned "the golden age of cardiology"—the last 40 years of the 20th century—an era that encompassed an exponential growth in knowledge and technology, as well as improved diagnosis and treatment of the cardiovascular system. The entire century was medically exciting, with the control of epidemics and pandemics of infectious disease by immunization, the development of the miracle drugs—sulfa, penicillin, anti-tuberculosis medications, and insulin—as well as, the elimination of smallpox by immunization, the suppression of malaria, and the discovery of polio and childhood illness vaccines. In the last half of the 20th century, quality of care was enhanced as medicine moved from an antiquated profession of generalists to a medical care delivery system that elevated the generalists, through residency training programs, to board-certified family practitioners. Specialists and sub-specialists were, likewise, residency and fellowship trained and became board-certified in their respective fields.

Along with progress came change, not all of which was welcome or understood. The public bewailed the demise of the friendly, but sometimes gruff and authoritative general practitioner who made house calls, delivered babies at home, and took out an appendix on the kitchen table; often paid for with chickens, eggs, potatoes, a smoked ham, or garden vegetables. He was "their" doctor and a trusted professional. His skill level in their eyes was dependent not only on his professional training, but also on their trust and confidence in him. My 90-year-old uncle, Kermit, recalls that when he was born at home in 1920, his mother, a devout and strict Christian, noted that the attending doctor had been drinking and was (?) mildly inebriated when he assisted in the delivery.

She accepted this, I am sure, in respect for his professional training, knowledge, skill, and reputation.

Medical practice is now perceived as being more impersonal and as a result the doctor-patient relationship has suffered. I have always tried to dispel that myth, making my patient encounters as much an interpersonal relationship as possible, hopefully reassuring the patient (never say "client") that I was deeply concerned with their health issues. It needs to be said, however, that today the American public has access to more highly-trained and competent professionals in the medical profession with more advanced diagnostic and therapeutic tools at their disposal, than ever before. The patient, the community, the nation, and the world are the benefactors. Hopefully, future generations of medical practitioners will continue to combine all that was good in the past with all that is good for the future.

As I reflect on my 40 years as a physician, I feel my experience has been almost surreal—an "out-of-body experience"—and I marvel at how this incredible and improbable journey came to pass. I have enjoyed the experience immensely and I cannot imagine serving in any other profession or trade that would have satisfied me more. It was never a problem to go to work in the morning, or for that matter, at any hour of the night, weekend, or holiday, to carry out my responsibilities. It was truly a labor of love.

A few years ago, while attending my 40th college homecoming reunion at Luther College, one of my classmates, a career clergyman, in casual conversation asked me as he might ask a fellow member of the clergy, "Where do you serve?" I had never seriously reflected on my profession and my life in those terms, but he was right. I had been called to serve my patients through the medical profession just as he had been called to serve his parishioners through the church.

I will try to give you an overview of my career, totally from memory, and not from any prepared notes or diaries (there are none). My purpose is not to embellish, but to document. I respectfully do not intend to be judgmental, but at times it may appear that I am.

These stories, hopefully, will evoke in the reader, emotions of joy, humor, sadness, tragedy, pathos, sympathy, and empathy. Medicine is often practiced in a very narrow corridor between life and death. You may sense the anxiety, tension, and magnitude of emotions, necessarily elicited by split-second decisions when dealing with life-threatening situations. Being able to see humor somewhere among the chaos and shear terror of the moment was often what got me and my staff, as well as the patient, through the day. You will be my judge as to whether I have succeeded in making the story of this improbable, incredible, journey interesting.

INTRODUCTION

"A long journey begins with a single step."

—Confucius

I was born on May 26, 1936, at a birthing house on Oborn Street in Waupaca, Wisconsin, delivered by a midwife assisting a general practitioner. My mother hemorrhaged profusely during the delivery probably in no small part related to my 10-pound entry weight. The prompt action of a newly-trained M.D., Dr. Christofferson, was instrumental in stemming the bleeding, saving her life, and providing me with a loving maternal relationship that lasted for the next 21 years. Hearing about the suspenseful events surrounding my birth may have, unknowingly, initiated my respect for the medical profession.

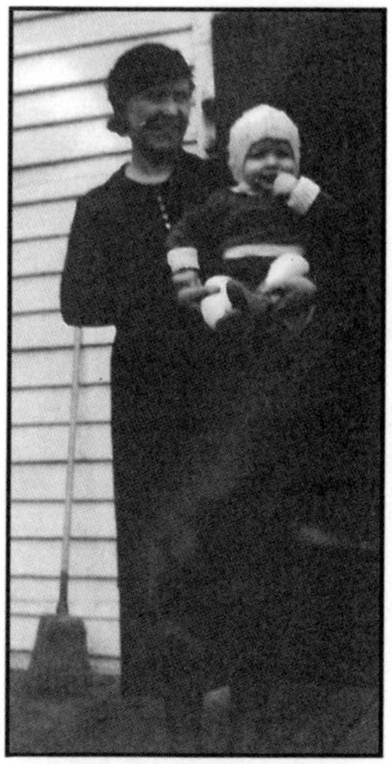

My mother and father and me

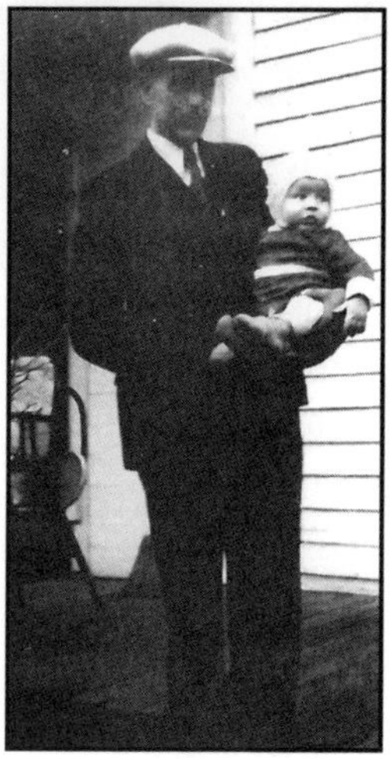

My mother-to-be was a schoolteacher in a rural one-room schoolhouse when she met, and after a two-year courtship, married a young farmer, James Peterson, on the Ides of March 1928. The Great Depression that descended upon the world one and a half years after their marriage made them very financially frugal and reluctant to have children until they were relatively secure. I was born eight years after the marriage. As far as I know, they came through the 1930s without debt. My father was very talented as an auto mechanic and machinery repairman, but he was also capable of doing electrical wiring, a skill increasingly in demand as the country began rural electrification of buildings and farms. For intertwined economic and family reasons in the 1930s, my father made his living away from the family farm where he was raised. In the spring of 1941, however, he returned to take over the operation of the Peterson farm. As luck would have it, farming flourished economically during World War II and in the post-war years. Although our life was very comfortable, farming never provided a financial windfall.

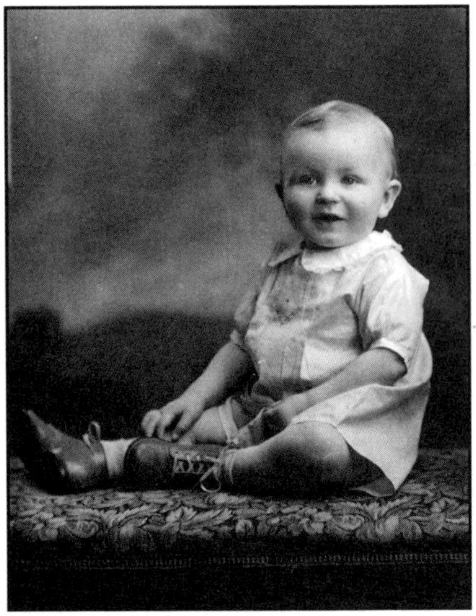
One year old

I'm sure my dad felt as uneasy as most new fathers, not being sure what would be expected of him. Like most men in the 1930s, he was fervently occupied with keeping his head above water financially, and I'm sure my mother and I could have easily become a second thought to him, but I don't think we ever were. The pictures of him holding me as a newborn, express a sense of pride and happiness one would expect from a new father.

Very simply put, as I was passing through adolescence and my teens, I began to know him as a most upright and honest man. I was influenced by his moral and ethical standards and by his uncompromising honesty and generosity. My mother told me of a time when he, while talking to friends, absentmindedly walked out of a Waupaca restaurant and forgot to pay the bill. He was devastated when he belatedly remembered his error. The next day, with gasoline at 25 cents a gallon and not to be wasted in his budget, he drove to town, apologized for his indiscretion in great humbleness and regret, and paid his bill. He didn't drink except for a rare beer with close friends and he didn't smoke. He didn't swear unless unconscionably stressed—I only heard it once—and the intensity of the impression it made upon me remains to this day. I idolized him and wanted to emulate his character but all too often came up short. When I severely distressed my dad with bad behavior, errant judgment, and even economic loss and embarrassment—I once destroyed his brand-new car in a stupid accident—he did not reproach me physically, verbally, or with sanctions. The fact that I had hurt him was enough for me to put sanctions on myself.

His mind and talents were genius, a fact that his unassuming demeanor hid from public view. On the farm he fixed the tractors and machinery and, unlike most of our neighbors, he rarely needed to take a major repair job to the implement companies. I have often wondered what my father would have done with his life if he had had the same opportunity for a college and postgraduate education I had. When asked in his last years what he would like to do if he had his life to live over again, he said very simply, he would like to repair used and old machinery.

Complementing my father's skills and personality was my mother, Gladys, who was very kind and understanding, always had a positive outlook, and had an excellent sense of humor. But, at times she could be outspoken, gregarious, and strict. When

Gladys spoke, Dad listened—as did I. As a somewhat rebellious teenager, I occasionally had heated arguments with my mother. She was the lightning rod and I was the lightning, or vice versa. However, I never doubted my parents' love for me, or for each other.

As a farm boy in rural Wisconsin, well away from any large or even medium-sized cities or towns, I was exposed to a lifestyle that was generic for this time and place. All of our neighbors were first, second, or third generation immigrant stock, mostly Scandinavian, exclusively Evangelical Lutheran, and extremely proud of their heritage and what they had achieved in America. I went to church and Sunday school every week, never missing a session in eight years. Along with my peers, I was confirmed into the congregation by oral examination at age 14, reciting Luther's Small Catechism from memory.

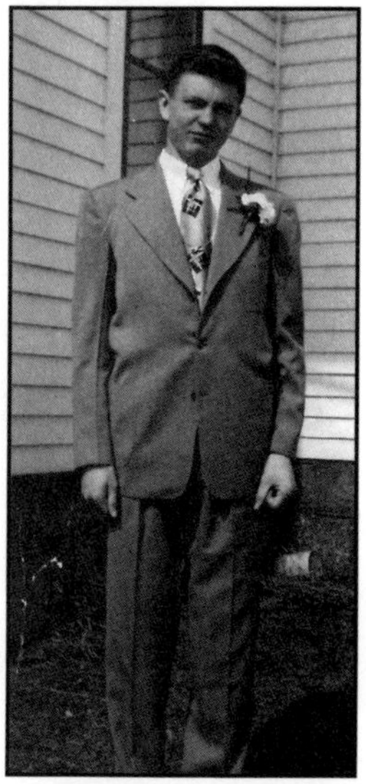

March 18, 1951, my confirmation at Farmington Lutheran Church

Like all of my friends in the area, I attended the one-room school down the road from our house called the Peterson Mill School. We spent eight years there repeating our parents' elementary experience: playing the same games at recess, studying the same subjects in class, and wearing the same style clothes—boys wore bib overalls, flannel shirts, and lace-up work shoes. We believed we were poor and by relative standards to bankers, lawyers, doctors, businessmen, and manufacturers we probably were. As children we assessed our wealth against that of our neighbors by the size of our farms, what brand and size tractor we had, or by what model and make of car our family drove. I now know that these were pretty inconsequential measures but at the time they seemed extremely important. I also know now, but didn't appreciate then, that I was richer than most due to my parents' love and encouragement. They controlled my access to the world, my friendships, my activities, my daily work expectations, and tried to teach me right from wrong. But, I was very strong-willed and often resisted many of their best and most noble efforts. This strong will, on the other hand, led me to want to excel at everything I did, whether in the classroom, during activities of daily living, or on the athletic field. Getting stuck in mediocrity was not an option and overachieving and thriving on competition motivated me to very high goals.

During my adolescent and teen years I was reluctant to discuss the idea of going to college because I assumed that we couldn't afford it. But, despite the fact that my education was not a common topic of conversation, whenever a decision about it needed to be made, my parents always encouraged me to continue in school. My dad was more interested in formal education than I gave him credit for. He was an active member of

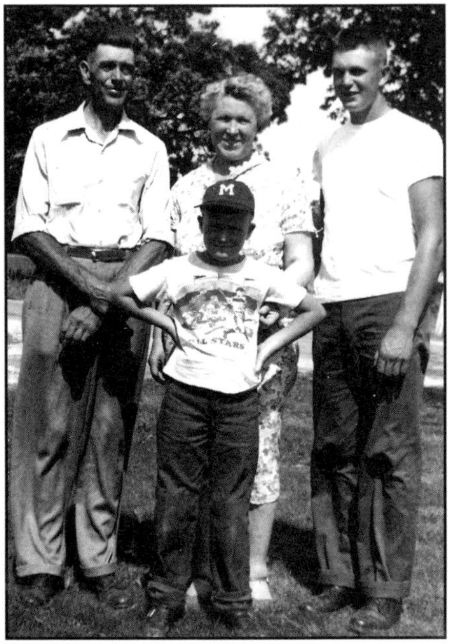

My father, mother, me, and my little brother Gordy

the school board for more than 30 years, often struggling with difficult issues, trying to resolve them in a fair and equitable manner. I'm sure my mother secretly hoped I would get a college education and travel a career path wherever it might lead. She herself had beaten formidable odds to become a primary school teacher. My mother was the seventh of eight children and the first girl after six boys. Her father, Charlie Terlson, owned a tavern in Hustler, Wisconsin, and was apparently a loving father during Gladys' early years. She was told that her father was so happy to have a girl after six boys that the whole town got drunk for a week on Charlie's dime. Of course, he may have just wanted to host a party and she was the excuse to do so. Whatever the backstory, Charlie became a much more difficult man over the ensuing years. What hardened his heart I do not know but my mother's next oldest brother in his later years described their father as a "rough old cob".

Immediately after my mother graduated from high school her father malevolently sent her out into the world to find her own way. Fortunately, she was befriended by some very kind people by the name of Gebhardt in her hometown of New Lisbon, Wisconsin. She paid for her room, board, and education courses—in what were called in those days, "Normal Schools"—by working as a waitress in the restaurant at the Milwaukee Road Railroad Depot. She also did housecleaning and domestic duties for her landlords, who I am sure, were subsidizing her generously. She would occasionally sneak home to see her loving mother when her father wasn't around.

My dad, by contrast, was the oldest of six children and received a very good formal education by the standards of the day. He attended Central Wisconsin College in Scandinavia, Wisconsin, in a commercial course of study following high school.

I'm sure my dad knew that if I received a college education, any chance of my returning to farming and assuming his role as owner and operator in the future would be unlikely. As was his nature, he remained quiet and noncommittal. I came to realize on my own and with the encouragement of my teachers that I was reasonably intelligent and adept, and therefore, they expected me to pursue higher education. But, I had developed very few goals beyond high school graduation. I considered getting a job or going into the military for a couple of years after high school before deciding yea or nay on college. When I told my dad this idea, he responded very succinctly with, "You better pursue your education while it is fresh in your mind." Those few words assured me of my parents' support and I knew that I would follow that direction, wherever it might lead. I'm sure that it was not easy for my folks to afford my education and we certainly never discussed the details of how it was possible, but nevertheless, I enrolled at Luther College in the fall of 1954.

Only two years later, my dad and I had to, once again, decide if this was the best course of action. It was decision time. It happened in the late summer of 1957. My mother was ill with terminal cancer and I was on the verge of returning to college for my junior year. I had to confess to my dad at that time that I was going to commit myself to a future in the medical profession because I believed that I really could do it and my professors were convinced that I would succeed. My dad pointed out to me that the farm we had developed and nurtured over the years was about as profitable and desirable as any in Wisconsin and that, as the oldest child (my brother was only 10 years old), it could be mine to operate someday. His words made a very significant impression upon me and made me more remorseful than any time in my life when I indicated to him that I wanted to go in a different direction. I didn't know whether I would live to regret my decision, but I knew it was what I wanted to do and I believed my reasoning was sound. My dad respected my wishes and, probably slightly begrudgingly, offered his full support. I know he was also concerned about his own legacy and the legacy of the Peterson farm for the future. When I left for college in August, I was quite sure my mother would not live to see me achieve my goals. I bent at her knee before I left and promised her I would not let her down or betray her trust in my abilities. She cried, and told me she had prayed for me every day of my life and she knew I would not fail. I said good-bye, feeling even more certain, with such strong support from my parents and with hard work, I would succeed.

Chapter One

BEGINNING THE JOURNEY

(1940-1954)

My early childhood exposure to the world of medicine was during an era before most antibiotics and vaccines were discovered and when infectious diseases were largely untreatable. I was immunized against smallpox, and have the scar to prove it, but no other immunizations were available. I was lucky to avoid serious illnesses except for a severe case of whooping cough that caused my parents to worry whether I would survive. Fortunately, I did not develop diphtheria, an upper respiratory and pharyngeal (throat) disease, which was almost uniformly fatal. Today, a trivalent vaccine, DPT, is effective in preventing diphtheria, pertussis (whooping cough), and tetanus (lock-jaw). I remember as early as age four being told that a neighbor boy, age ten, died of a ruptured appendix and a neighbor girl, age fourteen, died of juvenile diabetes. Streptococcal cellulitis (bacterial skin infection) and sepsis (blood poisoning) killed President Coolidge's son in the early 1920s after he developed a blister on his heel. My mother frequently reminded me to wear clean socks and to report any sores on my feet.

The discovery and use of sulfa and penicillin eliminated multiple life-threatening illnesses such as strep throat, rheumatic fever, scarlet fever, otitis media and mastoiditis (middle ear and mastoid sinus infection), as well as pneumonia. The widespread and sometimes indiscriminate use of penicillin to treat every respiratory illness, including the common cold, was considered to be a God-send and led to the near eradication of rheumatic fever and rheumatic heart disease—a condition described by a loquacious pathologist—as a disease that commonly "licked the heart and bit the valves".

In my adolescent years of the 1940s and 1950s, infantile paralysis (polio) epidemics were devastating worldwide, but even a single case in a neighborhood or community was frightening and led to cancellation of public gatherings, closure of swimming beaches, and strict isolation procedures. The most treacherous—bulbar polio— paralyzed one's ability to breathe, leading to confinement for life—often markedly shortened—in an iron lung, a primitive artificial respirator requiring enclosure of the entire torso in a tube-like chamber. In 1952, 658,000 cases of polio were reported in the United States, but with the arrival of the Salk and Sabin vaccines, polio was eradicated completely in the U.S. by 1979.

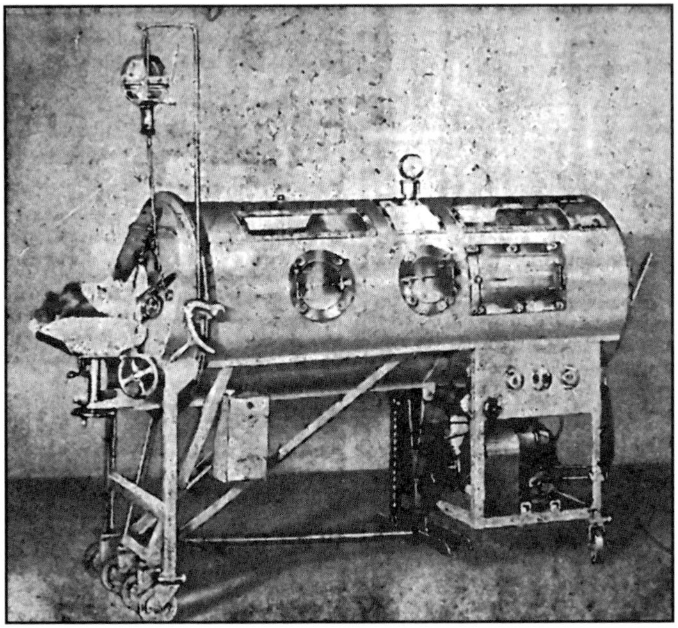

Iron Lung

Tuberculosis, a disease dating back to antiquity, was prevalent as a cause of death and disability up through the first half of the 20th century, most notably attacking the lungs where it could aggressively destroy tissue. The treatment often required disfiguring rib and lung resection surgery and the possible need for the Iron Lung; or it could lie dormant for years and then reactivate, spreading to multiple other organs. Cures were non-existent and return to a dormant infectious status rare. This scenario would change in the 1950s as anti-tuberculosis antibiotics were developed. A beautiful and vivacious young neighbor lady died of the disease after multiple surgeries and sanitarium incarcerations before these drugs were available.

Other more common scourges, German measles, red measles, mumps, and chickenpox were miserable to endure, but they could also be deadly. I remember each illness and their uncomfortable high fever and flu-like symptoms as if they happened yesterday. Confinement to dark bedrooms due to photophobia (bright light intolerance) with measles, the intolerable itching of chickenpox, or the painful parotid (cheek) gland or testicular swelling with mumps, could on rare occasions be complicated by encephalitis, a viral brain infection, leading to a threat of brain damage, seizures, or death. The quarantine officer, confirming the illness, and nailing a quarantine sign on the door of our house was never a social visit.

I was exposed to the medical profession in other ways as well. I often accompanied my grandmother Peterson on her monthly or bimonthly visit to Dr. Doersch in Amherst, Wisconsin, for illnesses real or imagined. My grandfather died in 1926, ten years before I was born, and reasonably, she was lonely and depressed. She would wait in Dr. Doersch's waiting room for two hours but her actual visits into his office usually lasted less than five minutes, which was time enough for him to check her blood pressure, pulse, heart and lungs, smile at her, and refill her pills which may have been mostly placebos (sugar pills or colored aspirin tablets). After these visits she was a different person, smiling and animated for days, but then the demons of loneliness and depression would slowly creep back. I was always impressed by the doctor's ability to perform this magical transformation with a few kind words and a smile. Whether I knew it or not, I was observing the art of medicine in the early 1940s in that small upstairs office above the drugstore on the Main Street of Amherst, Wisconsin. Dr. Doersch also would stop in at our farm on rare occasions to fly-fish on Peterson Creek. I would often go down to the "river" (as we called it) to talk with him for a few minutes. My friendly manner not withstanding, I'm sure my interruption of his rare recreational time was never too well received. But he never chased me away.

The biggest impression Dr. Doersch made on me was when he treated my acute otitis media ear infection. His house call, late at night in a blinding snowstorm with roads drifting full and nearly impassable, to administer to me and relieve my excruciating pain and fever, cemented my relationship with him and with the medical profession in general. After numerous bouts of tonsillitis and otitis and frequent absence from school during the first four months of first grade, Dr. Doersch performed a tonsillectomy and adenoidectomy on me at the Iola Hospital. Even after 68 years I have not forgotten that experience, but I never had a recurrence or loss of another day of school because of throat or ear infections.

The specter of serious illness or thoughts of mortality did not enter my consciousness to any degree until I was fifteen years old when a beloved neighbor,

Frank Carlson, who was relatively young and about the age of my parents, died suddenly of a heart attack. On the bright, sunbaked day of his funeral in 1951, I was left at home to "till" a field on our farm. As I walked barefoot in the cool freshly- turned soil, alone with a team of horses in an open field, thoughts went through my mind about my own mortality as I contemplated the sudden loss of Frank. That evening, I asked my parents if I could go to a movie as a reward for my day's work and they agreed. At the theater I noted that my feet were very sore and swollen from walking barefoot much of the day, stepping on chunks of dirt turned up by the tiller. The movie was, *Not As a Stranger*. It starred, among others, Frank Sinatra, playing the part of an idealistic young medical student who, after encountering egotistical and pecuniary motivated surgical professors, decided to move to a small community and join a senior doctor who shared his views about ethical delivery of medical care. There was a scene from that movie that remains with me to this day as vividly as that night in 1951 when I saw it. The old doctor suffered a heart attack, and Sinatra, desperate to save his life, opened his chest and massaged his heart. The sight of that open chest with the heart beating on its own and then gradually slowing and stopping as Sinatra is emotionally overwhelmed by grief is seared on my brain. The dramatic artifice of the movie scene overlaying the very real tragedy of our neighbor's death, made the psychological impression even greater. At the time, I might not have connected the two events, but in retrospect, this confluence influenced and directed me toward the medical profession and especially cardiology more than I knew.

Leaving childhood and entering my teenage years, I attended Scandinavia Union Free High School in Scandinavia, Wisconsin, a village of less than 200. The entire student body had only 55 students. In 1953-54, when I was a senior, I applied for a scholarship through Naval ROTC because I thought it was the only way I could afford college. I passed the extensive written examination in Oshkosh, Wisconsin, and then went to Chicago for a physical examination and an oral interview. The interview with a navy captain was less than stellar because I had not clearly established my goals for a course of study. Because I missed the last bus home I went to the railroad station to catch a late train back to Appleton, where my parents met me. I still can't believe I did this on my own. While waiting in Chicago's Union Station, I witnessed

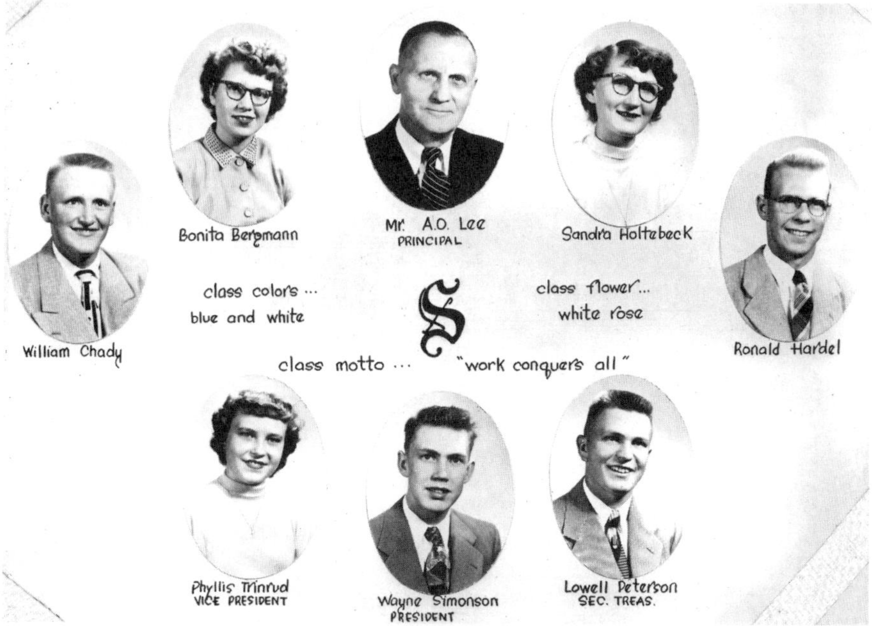

Scandinavia High School Class of 1954

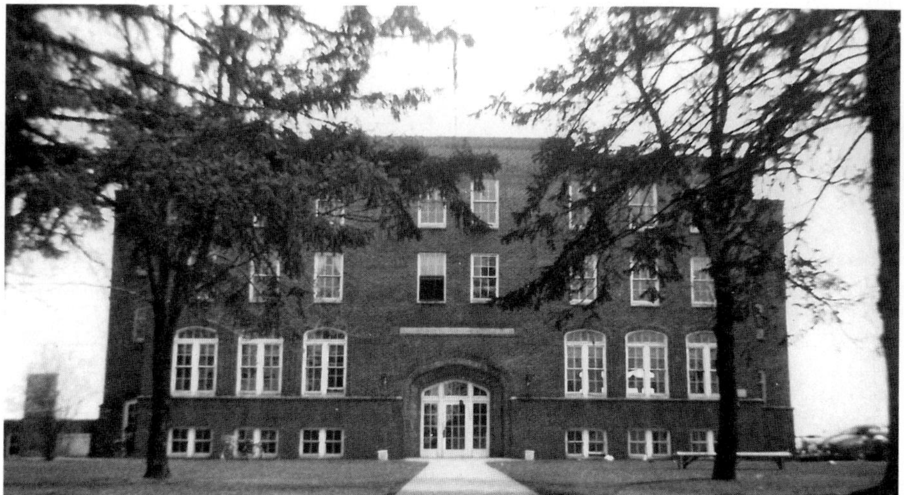

Scandinavia High School

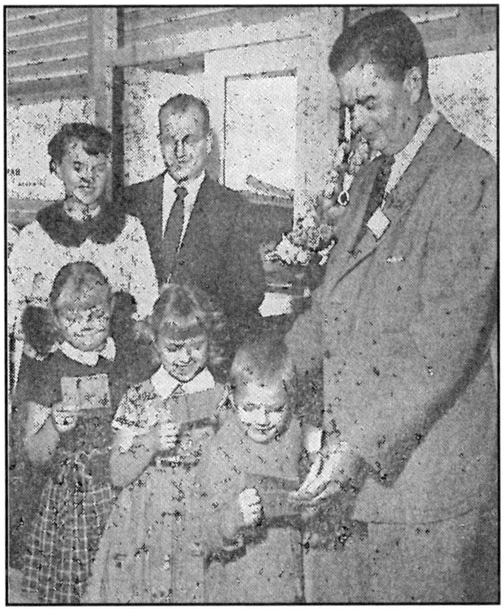

Dr. Klobuchar (right, with wife and family) indirectly influenced me to go into medicine. He was an Orthopedic surgeon in Green Bay before moving to CA

the departure of the President of Turkey with his entourage of security guards as they boarded a train bound for San Francisco. That was very exciting for a teenage country boy and it helped to take my mind off a long and stressful day. A few weeks later the navy contacted me and I made a second trip to Great Lakes Naval Base, this time taking the old North Shore commuter railroad from Milwaukee. I thought things went well, but after all was said and done, the Navy decided to deny further consideration of a four-year scholarship. Therefore, upon the urging and recommendation of my high school principal, A. O. Lee, I made a decision to go to Luther College.

I had no idea what curriculum or course of study I wished to pursue when I finally did get to college. I had considered teaching in high school, coaching sports, pursuing a military career, or returning to farming. One of my classmates and best friends, Wayne Simonson, told me he was planning to enter the military for a two-year enlistment, hoping to buy time and gain experience that would help him figure out his career path. He did exactly that, and after his two years of military service he also decided to enroll at Luther College. Interestingly, in that earlier conversation, he said to me, "Why don't you consider becoming a doctor? You are very good in science and have good grades." Wayne's uncle, Jim Klobuchar, was an orthopedic surgeon in Green Bay, and Wayne said I should speak with him about it. I did speak with Dr. Klobuchar and found his advice very helpful. Wayne also thought that if I decided not to stay in premed I could always become a science teacher, or use my science background elsewhere. Wayne also pursued that course for himself. He took college premed courses, was accepted to medical school, but found medicine not to his liking in the first year and dropped out. He went to work for a malting company as a chemist and remained there until his very untimely death in a car accident less than two years later.

When I arrived at Luther College and was in the process of registering for the school year, I met with an advisor who had been assigned to me. He asked me what I wished to study, and with butterflies in my stomach and my heart in my throat, I was barely able to utter, "I would like to be in premed." He promptly turned me over to Dr. Fred Giere of the biology department who helped me choose my courses. I was off and running, but where the path would lead, I did not know. I could only hope that it was not a quixotic pursuit of an imaginary and impossible target.

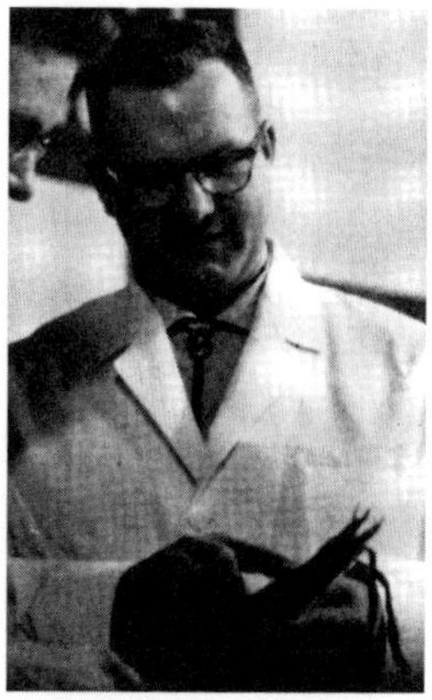

Dr. Frederic A. Giere

Chapter Two

LUTHER COLLEGE

(1954-1958)

Tucked within the rolling hills, high bluffs, and hardwood forests of northeastern Iowa, my alma mater, Luther College, a liberal arts institution, majestically overlooks the gently flowing Oneota River in Winnesheik County. The 19th century pioneer founders of the college established this center of Christian higher education with financial and student support from the large Norwegian Lutheran immigrant population of the Iowa, Minnesota, Wisconsin, and Illinois territories. Despite Luther's success and the relative prosperity of the surrounding community, the college town of Decorah, Iowa, remains to this day as it was in pioneer times; relatively small, rural, agriculturally centered, and not easily accessible. There is no train or airline access; very limited bus service by the Hawkeye Stage line; and the winding roads through the hills have only recently been connected to the modern interstate highway system.

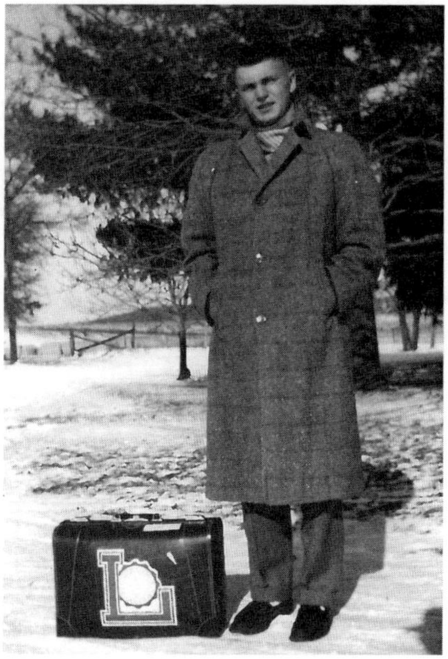
Luther College Freshman

Fifty-plus years ago, I lived 200 miles away from the college in central Wisconsin, and my access to and from school became an ongoing adventure. Although Luther College wasn't reputed to be a "suitcase college", nevertheless to some degree it was. The campus population noticeably shrunk on Friday nights as students scrambled to find a way home for the weekend. Only a few students had an automobile on campus. The lucky drivers had no problem finding passengers who would pay for the gasoline and the privilege of spending 36 hours at home. Those left behind had to find other modes of transportation. Hitchhiking was acceptable and safe for male students but the problem was, there weren't many cars traveling the rural roads of northern Iowa, southern Minnesota, and central Wisconsin. Still, my friends and I rarely gave our slim odds a second thought. On one occasion, my friend Wayne and I hitchhiked home on a cold night in late fall. After a long car ride with a deer hunter traveling north from La Crosse, we were dropped off in the village of Neillsville and the hunter proceeded on further into northern Wisconsin. We waited alongside the street in the numbing cold, trying to keep warm by doing calisthenics as we contemplated our misfortune. Finally, with the temperature approaching 20 degrees below zero, we were fortunate to flag down a semi-trailer truck. After we jumped into the cab, the driver informed us that his heater had failed and he was also uncomfortably cold. Forty-five minutes later we arrived in Stevens Point and caught the Greyhound bus to Waupaca. When we arrived in Waupaca at midnight we were quite sure we would find a neighbor, Inga Grove, finishing up her late evening waitress duties at Simpson's Restaurant and we could impose upon her for a ride home.

I don't know if public transportation options to and from Luther College have improved very much in the past 50 years—I doubt it—but it probably doesn't matter. The vast majority of current students have their own automobiles.

On the weekends we chose to stay at school—or had no choice but to stay—we still managed to venture off campus. Luther had very strict rules governing our free time. Attending dances and drinking, or possessing alcohol, were grounds for expulsion for one or two weeks or more. This was foreign to many of us, because we were used to attending polka dances, big band Saturday nights, and jukebox dance halls, where beer was served. This strict policy was a particularly unpopular temperance rule for the older male students who had just returned from combat in the Korean War. So, off we went to bars in Burr Oak, Calmar, and even La Crosse an hour away (the Avalon Ballroom and Shorty's Bar were favorites). One notable foray to La Crosse by Luther students was to see a new entertainer on his initial tour. His name was Elvis Presley. Using my keen foresight, I decided not to go, thinking that he was a flash-in-the-pan. It's not the only time in my life I've been wrong, but one of the most laughable.

Curfew at the girl's dorms was at 10 p.m. weekdays and 11 p.m. weekends, limiting the extent of social encounters. Most of the girls had their steady boyfriends either on the campus, or at home, so the pickings were slim. I had no girlfriends at home or at college, not by choice but by happenstance. For entertainment, I went to most movies that came to town and I forced myself to live on $10 per week, but after my freshman year, I would frequently exceed that.

As you might imagine, in the 1950s, at a Lutheran college located in conservative Midwestern Iowa, any color other than white would be unlikely. Our college was a homogeneous society and I don't recall ever wondering if Lutherans came in any other color. Maybe that is why I so vividly remember an incident that made me aware of the larger world around me. The Iowa Conference track meet was held at Luther and a big deal was made of it. The elected queen of the track meet had the honor of slipping medals on ribbons over the head and onto the neck of the event winners in Olympic fashion. This ritual was accompanied by a kiss on the cheek by the queen until one of the best athletes in the conference—a black man—won. His expectation and her hesitation was a moment of embarrassment for both, but there was no kiss.

I also remember a more personally sad comment on the times. A female Chinese student from Hong Kong, who in spite of being elevated to the role of Homecoming Queen by her female dorm mates, was subliminally shunned by the general student body because of her race. The memories of our conflicts with the oriental race during the Korean War and WWII were too fresh in everyone's memory. I thought she was a wonderful, upbeat person, and I couldn't understand how she coped with the underlying prejudice. In spite of being friendly to her, I felt helpless to do anything about her situation under the circumstances. As a result of the ostracism, she sought refuge with another foreign student from Germany, who I think was a closet-Nazi and hated everything American. I saw his influence on her change a very nice girl into a non-smiling, depressed recluse who no longer wore makeup. Looking back, it's easy to see that this was a graphic example of the times we lived in.

My social experience was less dramatic and arguably easier because I was blessed with friends like Ron James, who shared the back apartment of the Haugen house on 5th Avenue during my freshman year. He and I were different in so many ways but we shared a scholastic goal of success that college provided. We remained friends through our four years in spite of the fact that he studied music and was a terrific trumpet player, and I didn't have a musical gene in my whole body. That friendship remains to this day. Our other six roommates with the exception of one—Don Marquard, a Korean War veteran—may not have been as motivated. All flunked out, quit, or transferred to Mankato State in Minnesota after the first year.

In my sophomore year, due to the limited number of dorm rooms, I remained at Haugen's and roomed with an individual who was a religious fanatic and certainly not made in my mold. If he heard a swear word, often uttered by a Korean veteran, he would approach them and pull out his pocket New Testament from his breast shirt pocket and start preaching to them, pointing out the errors of their ways. I busied myself with my studies and avoided him as much as possible. When I moved to the dorms, as a senior, the counselors decided I could be a positive influence on my roommates and saddled me with the two most psychopathic of students. One was soon expelled for calling his religion professor a Nazi in an essay. The other was a spelunker who explored caves by himself—not too smart. As an example of his bizarre nature, he climbed the superstructure of C. K. Preus gymnasium in the middle of the night and connected a coat hanger with attached women's panties to an alarm clock timed to lower this item of clothing into the gym during the morning chapel service. Unbeknownst to him (maybe), a visiting pianist was performing during the chapel service. The convocation was interrupted by the perpetrator as planned and the undies hung above the gathered crowd for the remainder of the performance. The faculty attempted to identify the scoundrel who embarrassed the college and caused the student body to giggle. I knew there was only one person who could do this, but I didn't have it in me to turn him in. He was a genius, but a misdirected genius; I've often wondered what became of him; millionaire, Silicon Valley entrepreneur, or mental hospital inmate. Fortunately, during my junior year I lived at Dr. Gimble's house in a basement apartment with my hometown friend, Wayne, and Jerry Buerer from Clintonville, Wisconsin. It was the most tranquil of all of my years and we really enjoyed our relationship and had a lot of fun.

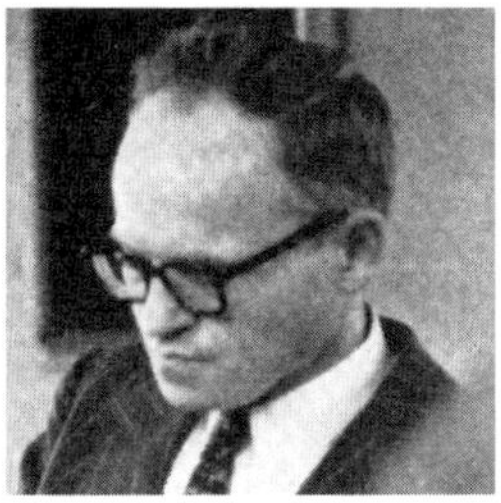
Dr. John Gimble

In October 1957, I was called home. My mother was dying. Her two-year battle with breast cancer was at its terminal stage. It was so unfair. She was a lovely Christian woman who deserved to live and raise her children and love and spoil her grandchildren. Cancer is a scourge of the devil and it is unrelenting in its lack of mercy for the good. My conscience tells me that I could have done so much more for her, understood her pain and suffering which were unbelievable, and told her what love I had for her. I failed in all categories, but at my age I was unable to accept the reality of the situation and I suppressed my feelings because of how much she suffered. My friend Wayne drove me home on Thursday night, October 3rd, and my mother died on Sunday morning, October 6th.

The year continued on a dismal note as the flu epidemic of 1958 did not spare Luther College. Most of the students became ill and were confined to their dorm rooms. Nurses, including Mrs. Hoslett, wife of my biology mentor, made rounds of the rooms daily, taking temperatures, checking vital signs, and prescribing medicines and nourishment needs. I was so miserable I thought I would die, but, along with all the others, I survived.

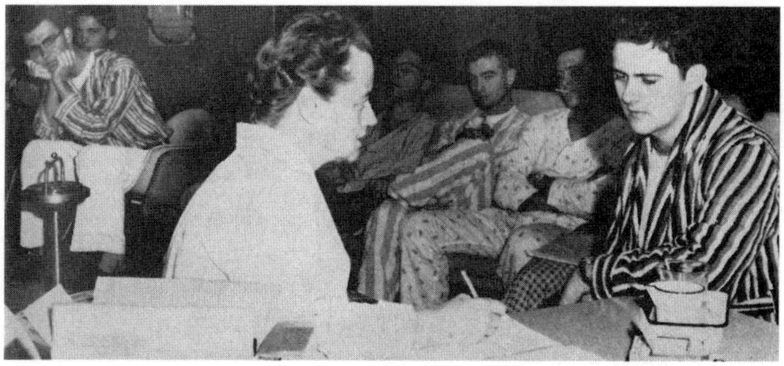

Photo from early 1958 Luther College newspaper "College Chips" *showing Nurse Hoslett attending to college kids with the Asian flu*

When it was over and I was able to attend classes and function again, I felt the need to go home for a weekend break. When I arrived, I opened the door. There was not a sound. The house was unlit and dreary and had a feeling of impending death about it. I walked quietly in, not knowing what to expect and found the hired man on the couch, my brother on another couch, and my dad in his bed. They all had the flu and were very ill. They had continued to do the farm chores with the aid of a neighbor, Osborn Gunderson, but they only had energy enough to do the bare minimums. I rolled back my eyes to the shock of the inevitability of my situation—college boy had again become farm boy. I made them all stay in bed and administered to them as best I could with food, drink, and medicines. I received the milking instructions for our dairy herd from my dad and I went to work. I was home for two weeks until they improved and were able to resume the farm activities. I fell behind in my studies as a result of this hiatus but I wouldn't have had it any other way. It was a matter of priorities and for once, this time I got it right. I caught up in my studies with the help of very understanding professors and dropped one class to lighten my load.

♥

I have a great deal of respect for the college and the education provided me, which is in no small part due to dedicated faculty members of multiple disciplines. There were some notable exceptions, who lacked emotion or interest in their subject, or were only interested in teaching students majoring in their subject. The most disinterested professor I had was a sociology teacher. His class was an exercise in predictable boredom. He always arrived in the classroom late, sat in his chair behind the desk and read aloud from the textbook for the next 30 minutes without making clarifying comments or bullet points. The entire class conspired to liven it up a bit with a behavioral experiment of their own. Before class we removed his chair from the room and made sure that there were no other chairs available. When the professor entered the classroom he stopped and gazed in wonder at the empty spot behind the desk. Without a word he turned on his heels and walked out of the classroom. Moments later he returned with a chair from another classroom and proceeded with his usual boring recitation.

Some teachers clearly wanted to educate us and see us succeed. Dr. Sherman Hoslett, the chair of the biology department was my primary mentor for four years, teaching me zoology, comparative anatomy, and histology. Other members of the biology department, Dr. Fred Giere and Professor Louise Ambuel, were also outstanding teachers and I remember them with great affection. Dr. Giere taught physiology and Ms. Ambuel taught genetics, general biology, botany, and zoology.

Off-campus field trips were a part of the curriculum. One of our most interesting was a journey to the Minnesota State Mental Hospital in Rochester, Minnesota, for the purpose of studying human genetic abnormalities. These conditions were of such severity that institutionalization was necessary. In addition to studying these individuals, a patient with tertiary

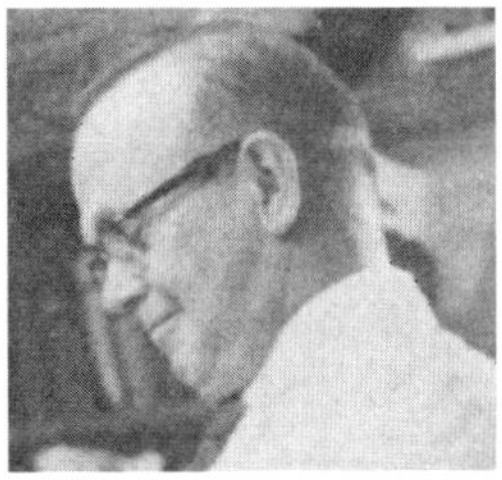

Dr. S. Hoslett

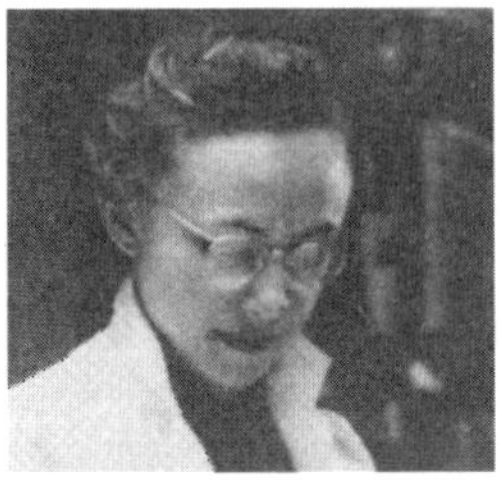

Louise Ambuel

brain destroying syphilis was allowed to speak to us from the auditorium stage for demonstration purposes. He had delusions of grandeur that were outlandish. He presented a monologue in such an entertaining manner that I could have listened to him all day. He stated that he was from a farm where each cow gave 500 pounds of milk per day and it was all cream. He sent his milk to the creamery in platinum milk cans and was paid in solid gold bars. His performance, psychotic and bizarre, was amazing and uplifting in the midst of an otherwise depressing presentation of the unfortunate individuals with genetic mental and physical impairments. Also, less amusing was a skull X-ray of a patient who had pounded a 10-penny nail into the center of his head without hitting any vital structures. There is little doubt that he was confined where he belonged.

My favorite type of study was more hands-on. While studying comparative anatomy, I was required to do a lot of dissections of various animals, all the way from crustaceans with their exoskeletons, to sharks with their cartilaginous skeletons, and then to mammals with their bony skeletons. The latter category involved the dissection of a large adult cat that had been embalmed and its blood vessels injected with red and blue latex. This may seem very gross to most people, but for me, it was extremely exciting and made me more enthusiastic about getting to medical school and pursuing the anatomical study of the human body. Because the dissection of the cat was very time consuming and required extensive study and memorization of muscles, bones, and internal organs, I elected to take my cat home with me over Christmas vacation. I packed the cat in the box with my dirty laundry. Needless to say, my mother was not too happy about this and made me take the box, cat, and laundry directly to the basement. I wanted to show off what I was learning about anatomy, and could not understand why she did not want to let me demonstrate my findings. I kept the embalmed brain and heart of that cat in a jar with formaldehyde solution for many years in that same house. If my mother had lived, I am sure she would not have allowed this macabre treasure to remain.

Lab experiments were sometimes too vivid, especially for the underclassmen taking biology as a science requirement for graduation. One of the experiments I demonstrated to a freshman biology class in my role as a teaching assistant, (T. A.), was the visualization under the microscope of spermatozoa swimming in a saline water bath. I was supposed to euthanize a rat, remove the testicles and fillet them, emptying the contents into the water baths in the small petri-dishes to observe the little squiggler sperm under the microscope. I arrived for the first hour laboratory session a bit late and therefore took the euthanized rat's testicles into the laboratory and proceeded with the filleting and preparation of the water baths with all of the students standing and watching. I had barely gotten started with the preparation when a boy in the group fainted dead away. I realized that, thereafter, all such preparation needed to be carried out ahead of time, not in front of the students.

In the biology laboratories we always had white rats that were used for experiments and demonstrations. It was the duty of the T. A.s to feed and water the rats and clean the cages. My fellow T. A., Russ Rulon, and I wore white lab coats and would occasionally take the very tame rats, put them in our lab coat pockets, and go out onto the campus with the rat's head peeking out. Because the biology laboratory was in the basement of a girl's dormitory—Larson Hall—we didn't have to go far to generate a good deal of excitement, much to our delight.

Adrian Docken, the chair of the chemistry department was an outstanding influence on me and he often allowed me to do extra credit work in organic chemistry. I recall making ethyl alcohol that was used in the laboratory as a solvent

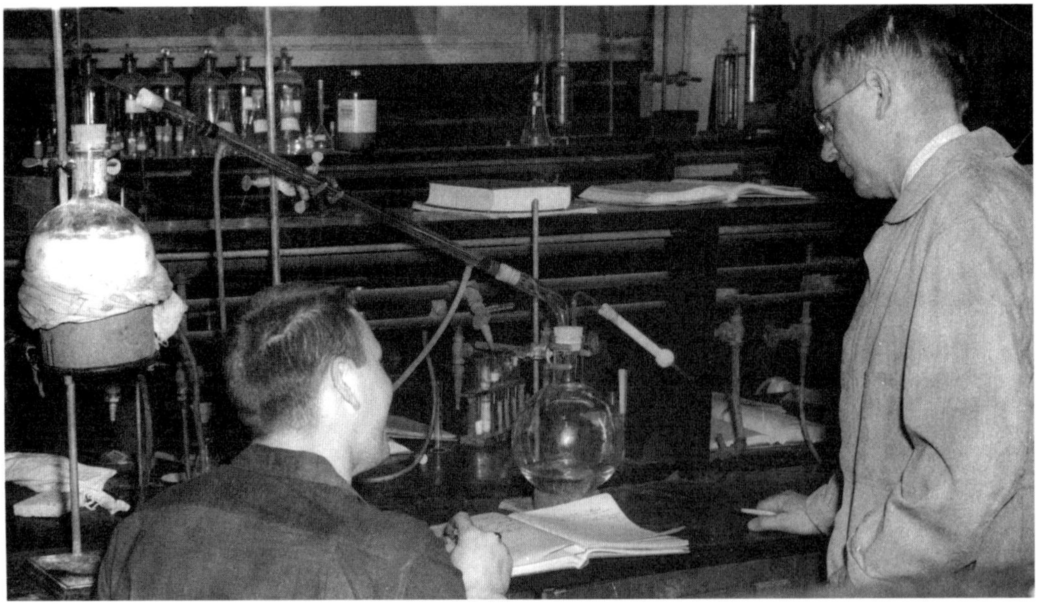

Dr. Adrian Docken critiques my organic chemistry experiment

for certain experiments. Therefore, on this campus that did not allow students to possess alcohol, I was running a "still" that would have made Appalachian hillbillies envious. On another occasion, I made soap, but was very disappointed that I could not find an appropriate hardening agent that would make it into a bar. Well, I have the distinction of having discovered liquid soap long before it was ever produced commercially, but I didn't recognize the significance of my discovery. It just shows that when fate kicks you in the shins you better pay attention.

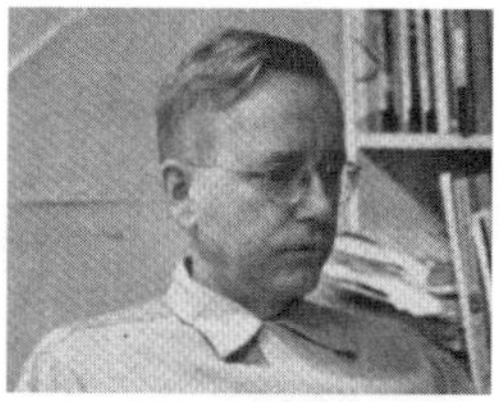

Adrian Docken

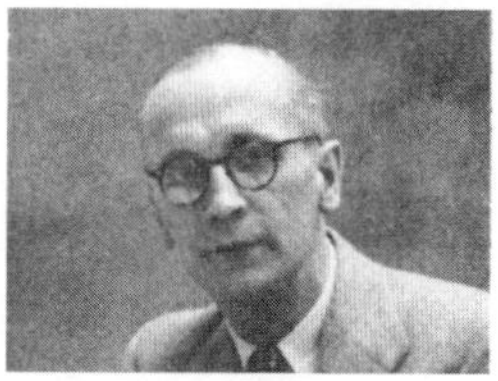

Herbert Rebassoo

Professor Rebassoo taught me college algebra, trigonometry, and analytical geometry, but I was able to sidestep calculus. He was a very nervous individual who would break numerous pieces of chalk at every session because he would hit the blackboard with such intensity trying to make a point. He was a refugee from eastern Europe after World War II and this probably accounted for his anxiety, impulsiveness, and chain-smoking. One of the main tenets of his teaching, simple as it seems, that I will never forget, is that "Zero is a number, it is not nothing."

In History I had the great honor of taking numerous courses from an extremely intelligent man, Dr. John Gimble. He handpicked several senior students to take a special course called European Intellectual History. Fortunately, I was chosen to join this class and probably for the first time was educated in how to think, not just how to memorize. We discussed the works of Adam Smith, Thomas Paine, John Stuart Mills and other great thinkers whose writings were the backbone of the American Constitution and the laws of this nation. It was a very deep subject to comprehend and I mostly listened in awe as the material flew by me—but it did make me think. I will be forever grateful for that opportunity.

Dr. Gerhard Belgum and Rev. Knute Lee of the religion department were dynamic teachers and taught me a great deal about history and philosophy as well as religion. John Helms was a superb young teacher of the classics and I was fortunate to have him as my professor of Latin. I had an excellent two years of Latin under Prof. A. O. Lee in high school that put me in good stead with Professor Helms. At the end of the second year of college Latin I was able to free-read the works of Cicero and understand them. Unfortunately, in this day and age, Latin

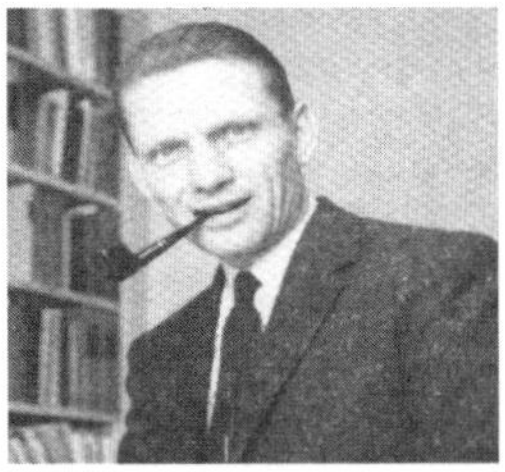

Pastor Gerhard Belgum

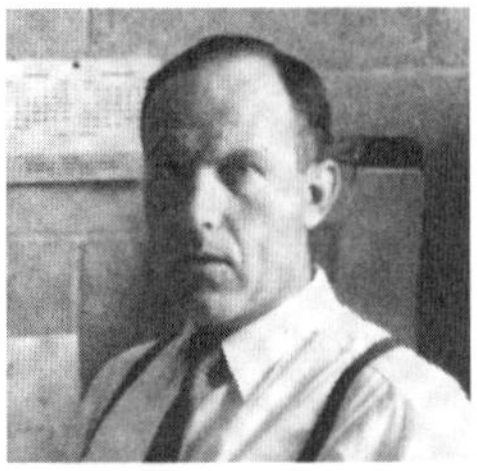

Pastor Knute Lee

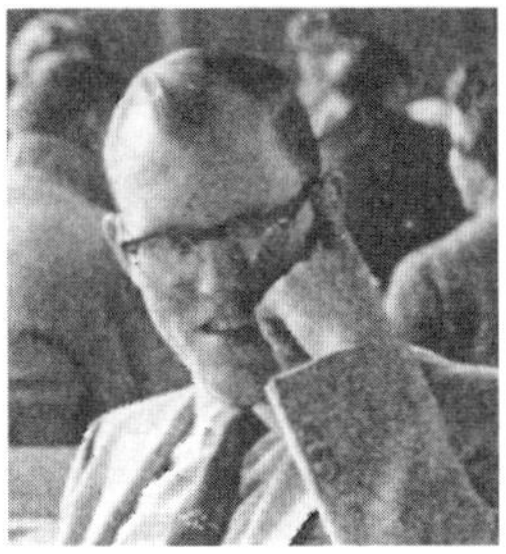

John Helms

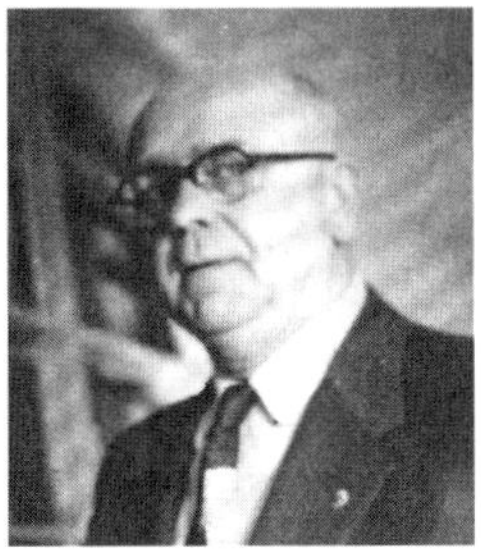

Dr. Chellis Evanson

is not as useful as modern foreign languages, but it helped me a great deal in comprehending and utilizing the English language. My son teases me facetiously, that it still might be useful if I happen to run into a Centurion on my way to the Forum. Another history professor, Dr. Chellis Evanson, stood in front of the window in his classroom and exhorted his class to become acquainted with that building on the other side of the campus. It was the library. He would say, "That's the book house over there; get familiar with it." Somehow the message got through and has stayed with me.

The Medical College Admissions Test (MCAT) is a very difficult exam of several hours duration testing the student's knowledge, not only in the sciences, but also in many other comprehensive subjects. A poor MCAT result is the kiss-of-death to anyone hoping to go on to medical school. Some students did not get into medical school mostly due to faults of their own. One individual who started out in premed and certainly had the intelligence to make it, progressively slipped backwards academically because he was on the football team. This required many late afternoon hours of practice throughout the week—hours that could not be spent in biology and chemistry laboratories or studying. It was sad to see. Another individual made it known to the people of his hometown community that he was going to become a doctor. He had poor work habits and lacked the caliber of intelligence that was necessary. He tried to keep up with his work in the laboratories by cheating, or what we call "dry-labbing". He was constantly trying to get the rest of us in the lab to give him information so he would not have to complete the work himself. This was despicable. It soon became obvious to everyone that this was the case and he was shunned. Thank the Lord and the powers that be, he never was foisted onto an unwary public as a physician.

The hard work and intensity required to achieve the grades and pass the exams to get into medical school seemed at the time to be incomprehensible. In my four years at Luther College, I observed students from similar backgrounds as mine, change majors, transfer to other less rigorous academic institutions, or just drop out. Far from these observations discouraging me, I persevered, and felt that I could keep going. So, in 1958, I graduated from Luther College with a Bachelor of Arts degree with majors in biology and chemistry and a minor in history. My dad came to the graduation, an endorsement of my success at college and the career expectations to follow. I think he was very proud, silently speaking for himself and for my mother. Little did I know what lay ahead of me, but I would soon find out that my intensity of effort thus far was not anywhere near what would be required of me in the next four years.

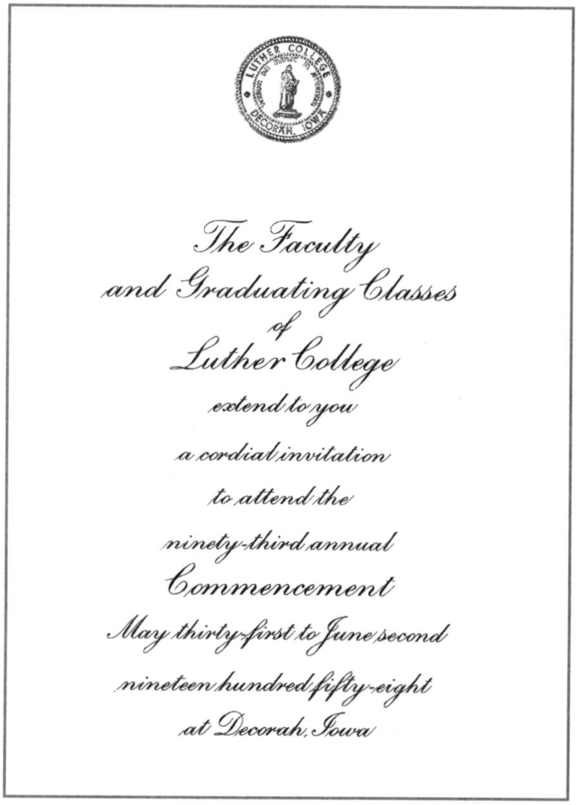
LUTHER COLLEGE
DECORAH, IOWA

The Faculty
and Graduating Classes
of
Luther College
extend to you
a cordial invitation
to attend the
ninety-third annual
Commencement
May thirty-first to June second
nineteen hundred fifty-eight
at Decorah, Iowa

Chapter Three

MEDICAL SCHOOL—THE FIRST DAY

(September 1958)

In mid-September 1958, I stood on the expansive front steps of the University of Wisconsin General Hospital for the first time, gazing upward in awe at the large stone building in front of me. I hesitated long enough to take in the panorama of the campus and felt a bit like Dorothy in the *Wizard of Oz* when she realized that she was no longer in Kansas (or in my case, Iowa) anymore. The giant metal doors in front of me did not seem very friendly or inviting, but nevertheless, summoning up what courage I could muster, I strode up the remaining steps of the hospital and boldly entered into a new world.

Each of the matriculating first-year medical students was given an appointment to meet the dean of the medical school on this, the first day of the school year. The dean's office, I was informed, was inside the university hospital. When I walked through the front door I was greeted by what could only be described as organized chaos. The large lobby was filled with patients being admitted or discharged, surrounded by a multitude of concerned family members. The secretarial desks were staffed by ladies who seemed overwhelmed by stacks of paperwork and the tedious task of completing numerous forms on a typewriter or in longhand. I was at a loss to know where to go in this maze. Fortunately, there was an information desk staffed by a kind, prim, gray-haired, lady who I guessed had been at her post for umpteen years. She graciously directed me down the east hallway to my right toward the dean's office.

The door to the dean's outer office was similar to all the others in that hallway, including doors to the offices of the hospital administrator, chief financial officer, and the chief of nurses. When I found the dean's office, I stared for a moment at the large gold letters on the door that simply stated, John Z. Bowers, M.D., Dean, University of Wisconsin Medical School. I entered with trepidation, trying to decide in my own mind whether all of these doors were trying to keep me out or invite me in.

The quiet waiting room of the outer office had a large desk, free of the cluttered papers I had observed on the desks in the lobby. The lady behind the desk was likewise neat in appearance and very sophisticated in her manner. After I met the dean I understood that he would not have allowed his secretary or her desk to appear any other way. She invited me to have a chair to await my interview. I felt a bit uncomfortable, thinking that maybe a coat and tie was appropriate and expected, but I don't believe I even owned a suit or sport coat at the time. Fortunately, my dress was casual and clean, my shoes were polished, and I was clean-shaven and sported a fresh haircut. I found out later that one of my classmates arrived for his interview after driving all night from northern Wisconsin after finishing a summer job. He was unshaven, unkempt, and barely able to stay awake. An upperclassman saw him leaving the Dean's office and remarked in astonishment, "You went in there like that?" I learned later that the Dean was a stickler for the appearance of his medical students and hospital house-staff. It did not bother him in the least to instruct them to get a haircut, polish their shoes, or get a necktie that did not have the last month's food spills on it. He even offered to buy a student a new pair of shoes if he could not afford them.

As my interview time approached, I felt the anxiety level rising and the perspiration developing. The facial expression of the interviewee exiting the dean's office didn't do anything to increase my confidence. After checking with him by intercom, the dean's secretary said to me, "Mr. Peterson, Dean Bowers will see you now." With knees weak and wobbly, I entered the Dean's inner office and closed the door behind me. Again, I wondered if this door was welcoming me to the medical school or if it would soon be ushering me out to some other endeavor.

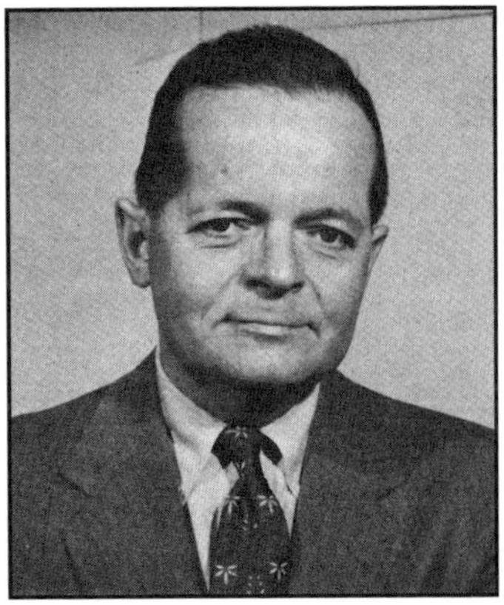
Dean John Z. Bowers

Dean Bower's appearance was stately and pristine. He was a stocky individual with the demeanor of bulldog sternness. His piercing eyes were only slightly dimmed behind his horn-rimmed glasses. He had a flat top crew cut that I was sure he never allowed to grow out. His long white coat was fresh and starched, covering an equally starched white dress shirt. His necktie was secured with a perfect Windsor knot, and his shoes had a military spit shine. Overall, his entire appearance and demeanor was that of a Marine commander.

To my relief, Dean Bowers rose from his large, leather, padded chair and gave me a welcoming smile. He extended his hand and graciously invited me to have a chair in front of his enormous desk. The first series of questions were ones I'm sure he already knew the answers to, such as where I was from and where I had gone to college. Digging a bit deeper, he asked about my motivation for entering medical school. I tried to be as honest and straightforward in my answers as I possibly could. I was never afraid to offer an opinion or state my position on an issue and I saw no reason to change during this conversation. I told him of my trepidation about entering the field of medicine without a family medical legacy as well as my insecurity about whether anyone with my rural background and small high school and college exposure had any business sitting here. I think he appreciated my honesty as he listened patiently, occasionally prompting me with further queries. I can remember very clearly his final declaration and challenge to me. He said, "Lowell, I think you will do just fine, and that you will become a good doctor and a credit to the medical profession. Just remember, keep your feet on the ground and your head in the clouds and everything will be okay." He stood up to indicate that the interview was over, shook my hand, and said goodbye. As I left his office, I suddenly felt confident about my chosen path. I would do everything in my power to never look back. Walking out of the building it seemed that the entire unlimited vista of my future lay before me. I exclaimed to the sky and to no one in particular, "Yes, Yes, Yes!" I was reminded of a children's book my mother read to me repeatedly in my pre-school years so long ago. It was *The Little Engine That Could*. As the little train engine commenced its climb of the mountain, it chugged out;

"I think I can. I think I can. I think I can."

The Little Engine That Could
Platt & Monk, publishers,
345 Hudson Street, New York, NY

Chapter Four

THE EARLY DAYS

(1958)

The vast dichotomy between anxiety and exhilaration describe the emotion experienced on my first day of medical school. I returned to my rooming house on University Avenue near Park Street and became acquainted with my roommate, a graduate of St. Norbert College, who was entering his first year of law school. We both cherished our affection for our alma maters but we would soon be acclimated to the cardinal and white of the Wisconsin Badgers.

The following morning I attended an all freshman class orientation at the Bardeen Laboratories Auditorium at the medical school. I was up early enough to shower, shave, get dressed in what I considered appropriate casual attire, and walk to the Rennebohm drugstore for a light breakfast. With pen and notebook in hand, I then walked to the medical school, arriving early so that I had plenty of time to find the Bardeen Auditorium. After reaching my destination, I sat near the center of the room as others began to filter in and fill up the seating. Our first-year medical school class had a total of 105 students, of which 100 were male and five were female (today, medical school classes approach or exceed 50 percent female). Just prior to the start of the presentation, a platoon of about 15 students showed up en masse, all dressed in suits or pleated slacks, blue blazer sport coats, white shirts, and ties. They walked to the front of the room and sat in the first row. I later learned that they were Jewish, had attended the

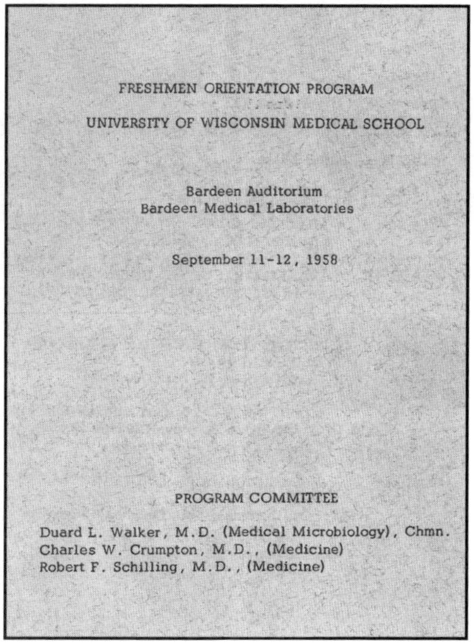

FRESHMEN ORIENTATION PROGRAM

UNIVERSITY OF WISCONSIN MEDICAL SCHOOL

Bardeen Auditorium
Bardeen Medical Laboratories

September 11-12, 1958

PROGRAM COMMITTEE

Duard L. Walker, M.D. (Medical Microbiology), Chmn.
Charles W. Crumpton, M.D., (Medicine)
Robert F. Schilling, M.D., (Medicine)

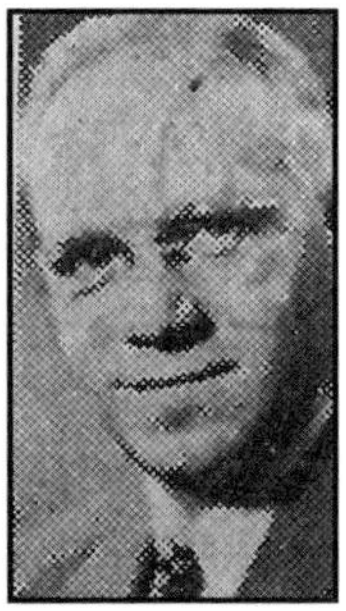

Dr. Mortenson

university in their undergraduate years, and were from Milwaukee, New York City, and the East Coast. They were obviously trying to impress the faculty, be visually recognized, and somewhat arrogantly, make a statement to set the standard for the class. Apprehension awakened in my soul as I reflected again on my rural background and casual dress. Did I belong here?

The presentation was given by Dr. Otto Mortenson, Associate Dean of the medical school and chairman of the anatomy department. Dr. Mortenson was an affable, father-figure type, with a full head of gray hair, rosy cheeks, subtle wire-rimmed glasses, and a ready smile. His soft-spoken nature endeared him to me, and these feelings of respect remained throughout my medical school days. I already had met Dr. Mortenson. It was his son, Peter, whom I had befriended during my junior year as a fellow student at Luther College. Peter had been kind enough to take me home with him to Madison for a weekend to familiarize me with the medical school and to research the admission requirements. I discovered that not all of my credits were transferable, and therefore, I could not be considered for medical school admission after my junior year of college. Although I was very disappointed, Dr. Mortenson encouraged me to complete my fourth year at Luther to expand my educational horizons and be even better prepared to enter medical school the following year.

In his introductory speech to our freshman medical school class, Dr. Mortenson advised us of "housekeeping activities" that were required in preparation for the start of classes. We were given handouts informing us of textbooks to purchase from the university bookstore, and arrangements were made for us to complete any payment of tuition or laboratory fees still pending. Dr. Mortenson also very clearly laid out his expectations and the expectations of the medical school concerning our ethical behavior in the laboratories, professional conduct with our professors, and respect in dealing with the human bodies (cadavers) in the anatomy laboratory. We would be paired up with persons of our own choosing to carry out the anatomical dissections, with two people assigned to the left side of the body and two people to the right. Horseplay in the laboratories was unacceptable and the bodies were to be treated with dignity. We got the message loud and clear.

Needless to say, I was not acquainted with my medical school classmates, and therefore I was at a loss as to whom I should join up with as anatomy lab partners. Fortunately, another student, Dave Zilz, a casual acquaintance in bygone high school years from the neighboring rural community of Iola, Wisconsin, spotted me and asked if I wanted to be one of his partners. He had attended undergraduate school at the university and, therefore, knew some of the other students. We soon put together our foursome. As it turned out, Liz Weber, one of the five girls in the class, would be my partner and Dave would partner with another student on the other side of the cadaver. Things were starting to come together and I did not feel as lonely as when I had walked into the room.

The afternoon was spent buying textbooks and the spiral notebooks soon to be inundated with mountains of handwritten notes from each of my class lectures. That evening, led by a contingent familiar with the bar scene in Madison, several classmates and I gathered to drink some beer and become better acquainted. At some point during the evening, I realized that our entire class was relatively small—just over 100 students—and over the next four years we would do everything together. We would study, attend lectures, carry out laboratory experiments, dissect cadavers, and take extensive gut-wrenching examinations together. Eventually, we would break up into very small groups and be introduced to patient care on the hospital wards. In other words, we were stuck with each other for better or worse. The following day the adventure would begin in earnest. At this point, not knowing what to expect, I satisfied my mind by just knowing I had made it this far. I was a medical student!

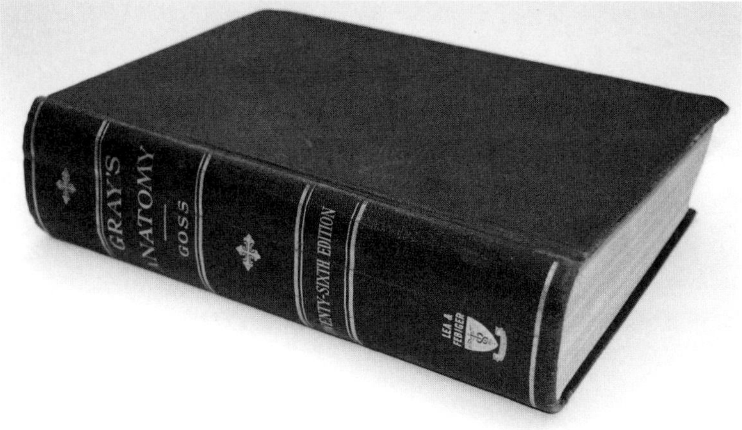

My Gray's Anatomy textbook, twenty-sixth edition, published in 1954

Chapter Five

THE FIRST TWO YEARS

(1958-1959)

The first and second year of medical school flew by so rapidly that I hardly had a chance to contemplate the speed at which I was advancing. It seemed that my time was spent in constant, non-ending study. Classes would usually end at 5 p.m. and, after a quick meal, I would study until 1 a.m. and be up again at 6, ready to take on another day. A Saturday night beer and pizza party at the Phi Chi medical fraternity house following a Badger home football game was a welcome break in what was otherwise best described as intense emotional and interrogative stress on a scale beyond anything I had ever experienced.

The medical fraternities had "rushing" events in the beginning weeks of my freshman year in an attempt to lure freshman class members to their society. It became apparent to me that most of the medical students that were married were in the Sigma Nu fraternity. The Phi Chi fraternity, on the other hand, consisted primarily of young single guys who liked to party when the opportunity arose. Pizza parties with student nurses from St. Mary's Hospital or Madison General Hospital were pleasant social events as there was otherwise very little time for dating or opportunity to interact with the opposite sex. I found the camaraderie and the social life to my liking and quickly committed to be a Phi Chi. At one of the "rushing" events I was warned by the upperclassmen to go easy on the "punch" that was provided because it was made from 100-proof pure alcohol pilfered from the anatomy laboratory and carried

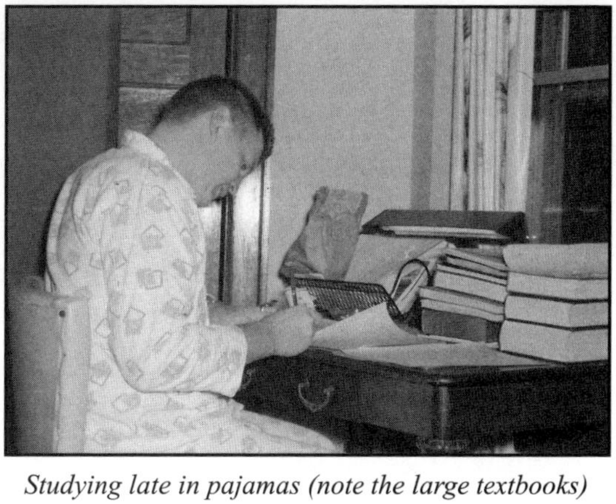

Studying late in pajamas (note the large textbooks)

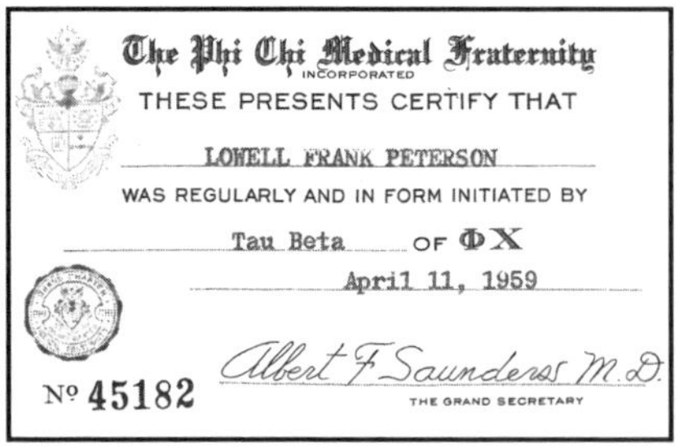

The Phi Chi Medical Fraternity
INCORPORATED
THESE PRESENTS CERTIFY THAT
LOWELL FRANK PETERSON
WAS REGULARLY AND IN FORM INITIATED BY
Tau Beta OF ΦX
April 11, 1959
No 45182 Albert F. Saunders M.D.
THE GRAND SECRETARY

back to the Phi Chi house in jugs inside innocent appearing briefcases. The custodian of the anatomy lab, who prepared all of our embalmed cadavers and placed them in alcohol baths, could be counted on to turn the other way while the barrel of spirits was slightly drained. After one too many trips to the punch bowl, not heeding the warnings, I suddenly felt very dizzy and became frightened when I could not hear the band. I excused myself and made a quick exit into the cool fall air, which fortunately worked wonders. From then on, I was much more wary of the punch bowl.

As I remember it, our first semester classes consisted of anatomy lectures, cadaver dissection and anatomy quizzes, histology lectures and laboratory, physiology lectures and laboratory, and physiologic chemistry (biochemistry) lectures and laboratory. I was immediately enthused with anatomy, both in the lecture hall and in the laboratory. I studied my *Gray's Anatomy* textbook, several hundred pages in length and about four-inches thick, in great detail. I also had a large atlas of anatomy that resembled a very thick coffee-table book, which I used in the laboratory to cross-check the pictures against my cadaver dissections for accuracy. The primary instructor in the anatomy laboratory was Dr. Antliff, a Canadian from Alberta, where he visited his large ranch on weekends via his private airplane. He was a stocky good-looking man who had also been a hockey player. During the course of our conversations in the lab I mentioned that I too had played some hockey, which I think helped soften his disposition toward me. (What I did not mention was that the only hockey I played was on local lakes and ponds with my classmates in grade school). Another factor working in my favor was my female lab partner whom Dr. Antliff liked to impress in a somewhat flirtatious manner. Our two lab partners on the opposite side of the table were not so lucky. For them he was unmerciful, criticizing their work and their knowledge of anatomy. He never hesitated to tell them that they gave wrong responses to his grilling, would make lousy doctors, and would not be a hero in their hometown. I felt sorry for them but I was in no position to be their advocate. I had all I could handle memorizing material for our daily oral quizzes. One of these individuals soon developed a serious illness and he was advised by the medical school faculty to drop out and not continue his medical school career. I don't know if the relentless harassment from Dr. Antliff was the cause of his condition, but I'm sure it didn't help. After recovery he entered the school of pharmacy, did very well, and eventually became the chief pharmacist at the University of Wisconsin hospitals. Another classmate—one of the phalanx of students who made the dramatic late entry into the lecture hall on the first day—also dropped out early on, probably due to the overwhelming academic expectations and his poor performance on quizzes and tests. Another student was requested to leave school later in the year after he had a psychotic breakdown and made a vocal outburst disrupting a class lecture. These situations were disconcerting but there was no time to dwell on their misfortune. I knew that the worst thing that could happen to me was to fall behind in my studies or let the stress overwhelm me because things moved so fast that I would have almost no chance to recover.

The histology laboratory for the study of the microscopic anatomy of organs was supervised by a doctor who played with the local symphony. He was clearly very intelligent and talented, but I found him to also have a priggish arrogance accompanying a belittling attitude, so I avoided asking him for help. Fortunately, his teaching assistants were more accommodating. Our examinations consisted of moving from microscope to microscope, identifying anatomical organ tissues or answering questions about what we observed. At Luther College I had not only studied tissues in a similar fashion but had also made slides of various organs by micro-slicing tissue, fixing it in formaldehyde, staining the slides with the H&E (hematoxolyn and eosin) dyes and studying them in detail. So, despite my aversion to the professor, I was able to do quite well in his class.

During the second year I was not as well prepared in pharmacology, primarily because I could not figure out during the lectures what it was the professors considered important and what they really wanted me to know. I did not do well in this mind-reading aspect of the class but I did enjoy the laboratory sessions, in which we conducted a few memorable experiments. One day, we had rabbits that were brought into the laboratory in cages. It was quite apparent from the beginning that whoever prepared the cages had not paid any attention to whether the rabbits were male or female. The entire class broke out in howls of laughter as the action began in the cages. I think that the saying, "rattle the cages", must have come from similar observations in times gone by. The girls in the class were embarrassed and the boys were amused by the observed promiscuity. Another (this time intentionally hilarious) experiment asked certain members of the class to sniff nitrous oxide, an anesthetic, colloquially known as "laughing gas". A classmate in my group, Walt Piering, was our volunteer. Predictably, red-faced, he could not stop laughing for at least 15 minutes while the rest of us were equally as exuberant in our laughing at him. In another experiment we learned the effects of alcohol on the brain. We were given grapefruit juice to drink but some in the group were given grapefruit juice with the 100-proof lab alcohol. Although we knew ahead of time that some would have the placebo of only the juice and others would have the cocktail, no one could tell by the taste who had what. Various tests were administered to all of the individuals to check reaction times and accuracy of responses. One of the girls got the alcohol and within a short time was clearly inebriated. As expected, her responses to the tests were bizarre, but the most interesting part was comparing her responses to those of us who only had the grapefruit juice—both were erratic. It was a great lesson in the power of suggestion and the placebo effect of medications. As I said, I did not do real well in this class, but the fact that I can remember these experiments would suggest that the class was not a waste of time.

In second year pathology, Dr. Lalich was very dynamic and instructive in all of his presentations. He was a hippie before we knew what a hippie was. His hair was somewhat long and he wore wire-rimmed glasses. He usually had a sweatshirt on under his lab coat and wore sandals on his bare feet. He would project slides of pathological tissue onto the screen in the front of the large auditorium and then he would pick one of us to come forward and describe what we saw. He expected us to describe in detail the characteristics present that would lead us to an accurate identification of the tissue and what disease process might be present. He would say, "Peterson, front and center; describe this slide," and I would do my best in front of my 100 classmates not to embarrass myself.

A humorous incident occurred sometime in our first year in physiology class. The professor, a kidney specialist who was scheduled to give a lecture on renal (kidney) function, entered the room, went immediately to the front of the room, and without a word began to write numbers on the blackboard. He wrote numbers such as, 2,920,000, 1,000,750, and 1,000,000. The "Gunners" (otherwise known as "Brown-Nosers") sat in the first row compulsively copying down every numeral before the professor turned to the class and said, "You want to know about kidney function? Well, these numbers tell you more about kidney function than describing the miles and miles of tubules in each kidney that filter wastes from our systems." (The gunners leaned forward in great anticipation). He went on, "The first number is the number of barrels of beer produced by Budweiser last year, and the second number is the number of barrels of beer produced by Schlitz, and the third number is the number of barrels of beer produced by Miller. I think that tells you better than anything else what the capabilities of the kidney are." The whole class broke up in roaring laughter as the gunners in the front row sat blushing profusely, embarrassed that their perfunctory diligence was so obviously silly.

And then there was freshman physiological chemistry, or as it was alternately known, biochemistry. These words alone still make me tense. I am not alone, I'm sure. I doubt that many of my classmates felt a burst of self-confidence whenever they entered the large hall for a p. chem. lecture. The head of the department was Dr. P. P. Cohen, who was ably assisted by Dr. Harold Deutsch and Dr. Salick. The latter was a very nervous, chain-smoking fellow who was very personable but who moved about so fast that it was like he was a cat on a hot tin roof. (Unfortunately, he would die of a heart attack at a young age). Dr. Deutsch gave the largest share of the lectures and they were so comprehensive as to be almost incomprehensible by those of us who had just entered into his kingdom. When I graduated from college I had a major in biology and chemistry but I was totally unprepared for the intensity of this course. Dr. Deustch would start on the left-hand side of the blackboard, and with chalk in one hand and an eraser in the other he would work his way across the wall, scribbling and erasing chemical compound formulas and biochemical pathways, while steadily explaining as he went. He never missed a double bond in his formulas or an enzyme or coenzyme on the pathways. When he reached the right end of the blackboard he would double back and start over, writing and erasing, talking and explaining. This would go on for an hour. All of these chemical formulas and pathways were combined together on a very large chart we were required to purchase and commit to memory. It looked like a map of the world with every town and city included. There was the entire pathway for the metabolism of glucose ending in the Krebs cycle; protein pathways ending in the uric acid cycle; hormone formulas and pathways; and other exotic metabolic pathways. Liz, my lab and study partner had worked for Dr. Salick as a medical technologist and she was quite knowledgeable about this complicated subject. I asked her if I was expected to know all of what Dr. Deutsch was trying to teach us at the blackboard as well as what was on the biochemical chart. She informed me in no uncertain terms that, yes, I would be expected to memorize all of it and be required to write it out on an examination just as he had done on the blackboard. I have never, before or since, studied so hard and memorized so much as I did in this course over that semester. The final exam was four hours long and consisted of regurgitating these formulas and pathways onto paper. A typical question at the top of the page would be "Show the metabolic pathway of glucose from the beginning on through the Krebs cycle recording all enzymes, coenzymes, pathways, and reverse pathways." The rest of the page was blank. I wrote without pause for the entire four hours. Nevertheless, I apparently missed an occasional double bond, enzyme or coenzyme, and did not do as well with the complicated formulas and pathways for the hormones. I felt grateful to receive a "C" grade in the course. One of my classmates arrived for the examination, sat down and wrote his name on the top of the paper, scanned the questions, and got up and walked out of the room leaving his paper behind. He went to the University of Minnesota and took the course again during the following summer and was able to pass it. He was allowed to continue in medical school at the University of Wisconsin the following year. Although I was elated to discover reserves of focus and discipline that I didn't know I had, I never wanted to face such a stressful experience again.

I learned a great deal in the classroom—about medicine and myself. But, one of the most important lessons I learned occurred one night in the beginning of my freshman year. I had an opportunity to attend a Big-10 boxing match featuring the top-rated boxer for the university. I always enjoyed listening to boxing matches on the radio in the 1940s and watching them on television in the 1950s. I was a great fan of Joe Louis and Sugar Ray Robinson, and later, Jersey Joe Walcott, Rocky Marciano, and Ingemar Johannsen. Watching the event at Camp Randall field house was a totally new experience. At a key moment, the UW star let his guard down and was knocked to the canvas with a sharp hook to the side of his head. He got up briefly but then collapsed and was taken to the locker room unconscious on a stretcher. As I walked away from the field house that night, I heard the eerie siren of an ambulance echoing through the night air and was overcome with a horrible sick feeling in my stomach. Being very unnerved and seeking solace, I decided to stop at Liz's apartment on the second floor of a rooming house she shared with Mary Danke. They were both on-call as medical technologists for the hospital blood bank and it was not long after I arrived that the phone rang and their services were requested for an acute emergency. I accompanied them to the blood bank certain that the patient would be the boxer and I was soon informed that I was correct. I watched as they cross-matched donor blood to match the patient's blood type. The chief of neurosurgery, Dr. Javid, had the young man in the operating room very rapidly, proceeding with the craniotomy (a large open flap-like retracted section of the skull to expose the brain and treat the traumatic injury.) There were no CT scans or MRIs in those days to assess the degree of injury. The surgery went on and on, far into the night and the early morning hours of the next day. Extensive hemorrhaging was emanating from the venous structures inside the skull loose in multiple places by the hard blow. Because of the extensive hemorrhage, numerous blood transfusions were required and I was pressed into service to deliver the pints of blood from the blood bank to the operating room. New blood donors were brought in but even with the infused fresh blood the bleeding did not stop. The situation became hopeless and the young man died. The sickening feeling I had in my stomach earlier returned, but this time it was accompanied by a heavy sadness and grief. A great stir erupted on the campus and in the press during the following week, with the public crying for boxing to be eliminated as a collegiate sport. A very prominent university surgeon and former boxer for the university, Dr. Anthony Curreri, fought very hard to maintain the status quo, but to no avail. Boxing was banned at the university and throughout the entire Big-10 Conference.

As tragic as the young man's death was, and as intense as the emotions were, I realized that I had witnessed one of the acutely stressful situations doctors are exposed to on a daily basis. Although I was an inexperienced medical student, my adrenaline was flowing, and I knew that I wanted to be in a position to make hard decisions and carry out procedures that could be lifesaving. For the first time, I also realized that not every effort, no matter how skilled the doctor, would always be successful. But I felt confident that in the future, I could deal with life and death decisions and face them head-on.

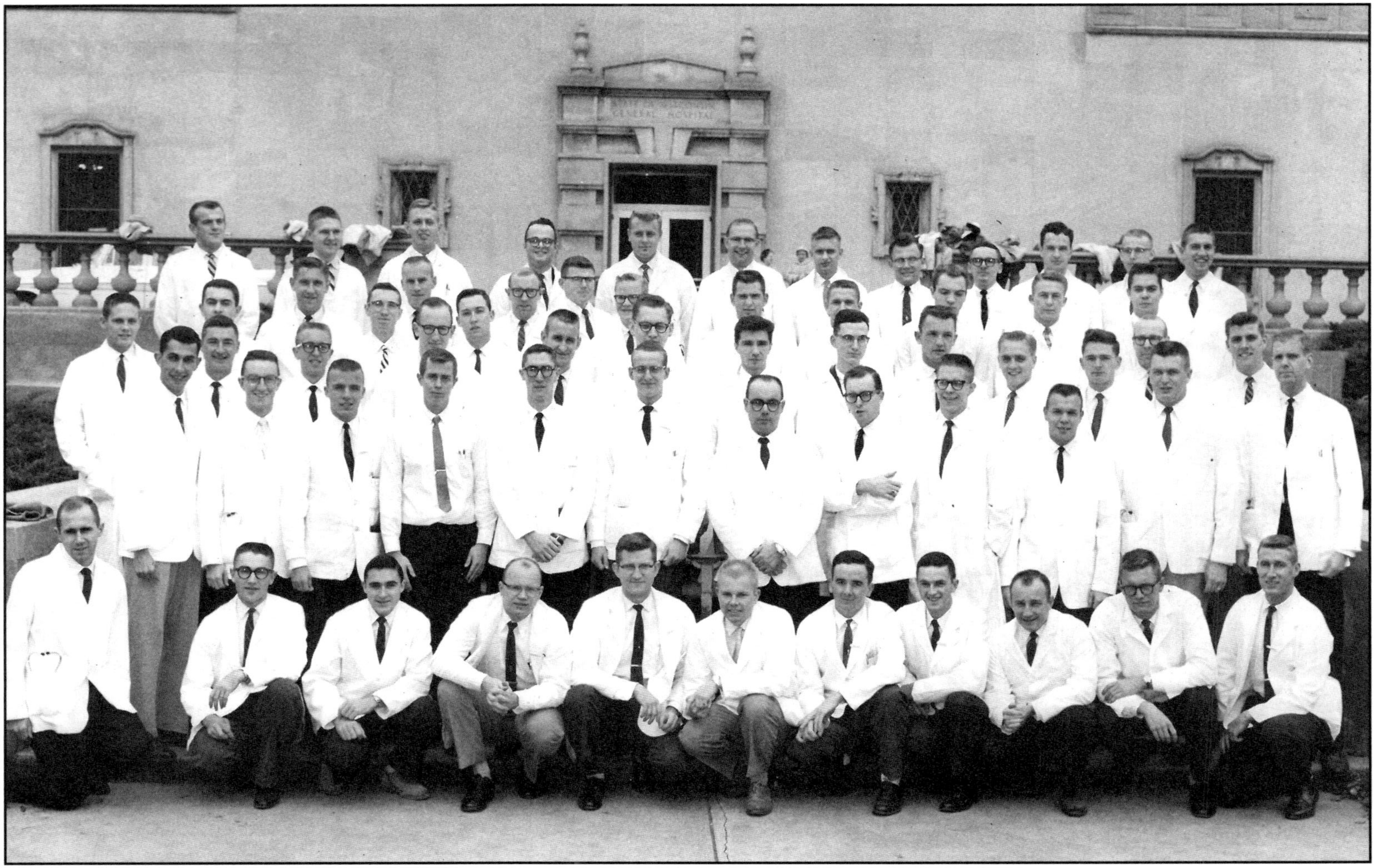

Phi Chi members of the junior and senior medical school classes. I am in the second row, second from the right.

Chapter Six

THE CLINICAL YEARS

(1960-1962)

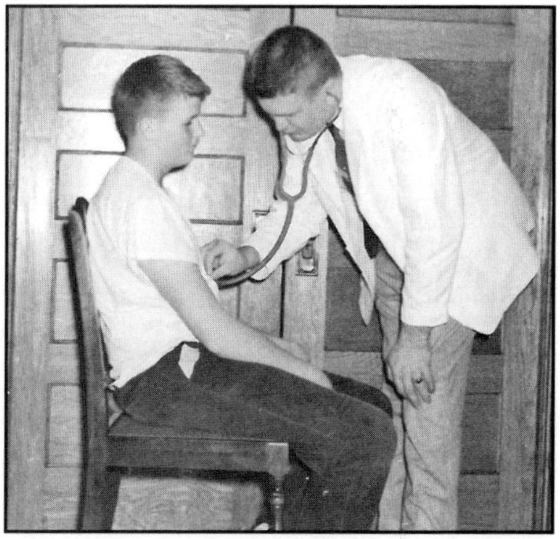
Practicing a physical exam on my brother, Gordy

Between the first and second year of medical school I resumed my usual summer college vacation routine of working on the family farm, playing baseball with the local town team, and occasionally carousing at bars and dance halls with my friends. This summer, however, I added another activity: assisting surgeons at the Waupaca and Iola hospitals. I asked the operating room nurses to call me whenever they scheduled a surgery so that I could "scrub in", and fortunately they agreed. Even better, the local general practitioners and the visiting specialists from Appleton and Neenah were more than willing to teach and, I suspect, more than happy to have an extra pair of hands to assist them. It was an invaluable introduction to the operating room and to a multitude of various procedures without the distraction of a critically observing professor. On one occasion a pair of GPs doing a gallbladder operation, finished the gallbladder removal and walked out of the room, telling me to close the belly, which of course I had never done. They were laughing in the hallway as they observed my panic. Merna, the seasoned and experienced nurse, finally took charge and said she would assist me and tell me what to do. I closed the abdomen in layers with running stitches and well-tied square knots that met with her approval. I'm sure the patient never found out that she had been sutured back together by a first-year medical student. This wonderful summer hiatus would be my last because the second year of medical school would continue right into the third and fourth without a vacation break.

My third year of medical school began in the early summer of 1960. I was expected at all times to wear a jacket length white coat, a shirt and tie, dress trousers, and polished shoes. A newly purchased stethoscope curled into the right side coat pocket while a pen, penlight, and tongue blades adorned my left breast pocket. A nametag identified me to my professors and to the patients. Most impressively, I carried a newly purchased crisp black leather bag. Inside were all of the instruments I required: an otoscope-ophthalmoscope for checking ears and eyes, a rubber hammer to check reflexes, a tuning fork for hearing evaluation and vibratory sensation tests, safety pins and cotton tip applicators for checking sharp and light touch sensations, a sphygmomanometer for checking blood pressures, and a small concise three-ring notebook that contained an outline for conducting and recording the history and physical examination. This notebook also contained charts of normal laboratory values and other vitally important measurements that I was expected to know. Overall, I looked—and felt—pretty professional, which I admit gave me a little jolt of confidence. I would soon realize, however, that a white coat and a black bag did not make me a doctor.

Although the strictly didactic and laboratory work of the first two years was over and the large textbooks of anatomy, physiology, pharmacology, biochemistry, pathology, and microbiology were put on the shelves, my clinical experience on the hospital wards with real patients during the third year would be shared with further didactic lectures and even larger textbooks. In the physical diagnosis class, taught by Dr. Leroy Sims, my classmates and I were divided alphabetically into groups of five and instructed how to examine hospital patients and how to carefully observe and record normal as well as abnormal findings. My group consisted of Clark Olson, Jerry Petasnick, Walter Piering, and Kathy Pizialli.

The first patient we evaluated was a 16-year-old boy with Hodgkin's disease, a malignant condition of the lymphatic system. Making the diagnosis was not difficult because he told us what his illness was, but I still needed a textbook to study this disease in detail. The boy was undergoing chemotherapy, a treatment still in its infancy, and its effects were brutal. Infusions of nitrogen mustard wracked him with nausea and vomiting and he lost all of his hair. He appeared old, anemic, and pale. I was shocked by his appearance and I felt guilty that I might be taxing him further as my group transcribed his medical history and fumbled our way through his physical examination. My classmates and I kept our emotions in check, but it wasn't easy. We kept our minds clear by concentrating on asking the right questions and staying attentive to the task at hand. After meeting with this young man, each member of the group had to write out the complete history and physical which, for the sake of completeness, was extremely lengthy. I felt that I had performed my duties well by dutifully submitting a thorough report. Each of our group was soon disabused of this notion when we met with the medical resident who fiercely critiqued our work. No matter how complete I thought the profile was, I realized that at this stage in my training I still had a lot to learn. As I was given the opportunity to examine more patients I began to feel confident in my ability to conduct a thorough, efficient, comprehensive history and physical examination.

My group also rotated through multiple other medical specialty services and traveled to nearby hospitals: the Veterans Administration Hospital, St. Mary's Hospital, Madison General Hospital, and the Mendota State Hospital for the mentally ill. Each hospital offered different case studies for our group to consider, but even more educational were the brief glimpses we had into other people's daily lives. A field trip to Southern Colony, a hospital for mentally and physically challenged children who had genetic illnesses (i.e. Down's syndrome, Muscular Dystrophy etc.), birth defects, and severe cerebral palsy was eye opening and left me feeling depressed. Likewise, field trips to the state schools for both male and female juvenile inmates who had been repeatedly in trouble with the law made me feel both grateful for my family background and saddened that I could not change anything in their lives. Trips to industrial facilities to become familiar with industrial medicine and work-related injuries and illnesses included visits to Allis-Chalmers Corporation and Oscar Mayer meat packing company.

One field trip the class a year ahead of us took was to the Waupun State Prison to observe the medical care provided to prisoners often condemned to this facility for life. In addition, this facility incarcerates the criminally insane. These inmates are often violent and unpredictable. Mass murderers, grave robbers, murderers who dismember their victims, and many other ghoulish criminal perpetrators are confined in this facility. Some of my fraternity brothers described one of the individuals as an insane albino who ate everything he could get his hands on.

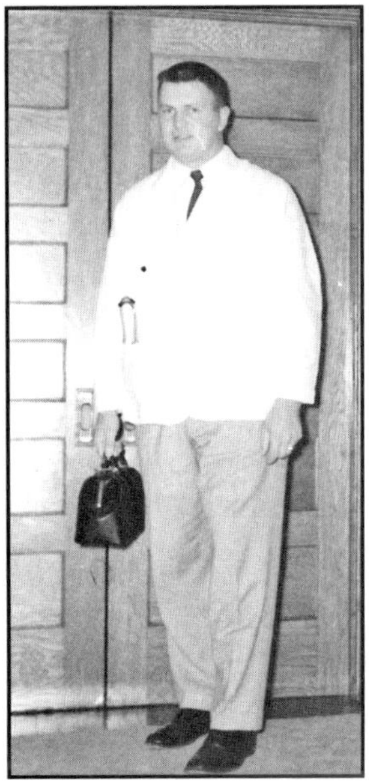

He was fed on paper plates, which he devoured along with his food. He had been given a small Christmas tree for his cell, which he promptly ate. Listening to these tales, I had a hard time imagining what it was like for the staff doctors to provide humane medical care to these inmates.

I had an excellent rotation through the obstetrics (OB) and gynecology (GYN) service both at the University Hospital and at Madison General Hospital. I delivered more than 30 babies while being observed by the staff doctors, most notably Dr. Bob Jackson and Dr. John Ellis. On occasion, the attending doctor was late in arrival for the delivery and the expectant mother was not about to wait. It was during one of these precipitous deliveries at Madison General Hospital that I met my future wife, an OB nurse. She talked me through the delivery, and I caught the slippery infant in my large hands. I looked over my shoulder to see who this kind and knowledgeable person was. A couple of weeks later, after we became better acquainted, I invited her to the movies. She agreed, although she probably didn't appreciate my choice, which was *The Guns of Navarone*.

My rotation in pediatrics was less memorable because I knew from the beginning that I did not want to follow this path in medicine. Why? It was simply heartbreaking to see sick children with cancer, leukemia, or other terminal diseases. Of course, in private practice, pediatricians see predominantly well children or those with minor self-limiting illness. Nevertheless, it did not appeal to me. However, there are two cases that still stand out in my memory.

The first was a rather unusual incident involving a 10-year-old boy who, while at school, inhaled a straight pin he was holding between his lips. His teacher immediately sent him home to his family farm, but when he arrived he found that no one was home. The boy then saddled his pony and rode it to the neighboring farms until he found his mother. She quickly brought him to the University Hospital where an X-ray clearly showed the straight pin was lodged in the left lower lobe of his lungs. He was not in any distress other than being frightened. The pediatric resident, in his wisdom, raised the hospital bed and had the boy hang his head over the edge down to the floor, and strapped him in place. Periodically he was slapped on the back throughout the night. In the morning the boy was coughing almost continuously as if he had a tickle in his throat. The morning X-ray showed that the straight pin had traveled to his upper trachea just below his vocal cords. An ear, nose, and throat doctor sedated him and used a laryngoscope and forceps to extract the pin. He was sent home later that day. I don't know if this course of action was one that the resident had seen before or if it was something he concocted on his own, but it made quite an impression on me. I saw how common sense and patience could resolve even difficult situations and that not all required heroic and grandiose interventions.

The other pediatric case was more dramatic and difficult to witness. I followed a young boy on the orthopedic service who was going to have a biopsy of a tumor on his femur, just above the knee. I asked the orthopedic professor if I could scrub-in on the case, and he graciously agreed. I was not well prepared for the gravity of the situation, however. It was explained to the boy and his parents that if the tumor was malignant the leg should be amputated. As the boy reached the operating room, he was crying huge tears and screaming, "Please don't take my leg off!" He was given anesthesia and the surgery began, with the surgeons making a limited incision and taking a biopsy. In due time, the pathology laboratory reported their findings from the frozen sections taken from the tumor, diagnosing it as a Ewing's Sarcoma, a highly malignant and lethal bone tumor that can occur on any bone in the body. (A neighbor girl of mine had recently died from a similar tumor on her rib). Hearing this damning information, I knew that only a single therapeutic choice remained; amputation of the boy's leg. I had a hard time dealing with this emotionally, but it helped me begin to understand the necessity of separating sympathy from empathy and proceeding with what is medically necessary.

Navigating each case, both empirically and emotionally, proved a steep learning curve for everyone in my class during these clinical years. Also difficult for me to reconcile, however, was my idealized view of medicine—one in which all doctors were basically the same: educated, highly-talented, ethical, respected, and superb diagnosticians as they followed the facts and acted nobly—and the unvarnished reality of daily life where I began to see them as human beings, faced on a daily basis with the frenzied battle against disease, with human frailties like everybody else.

When I was a senior student I was assigned to the thoracic surgery service of Dr. Joseph Gale, a gray-haired, rotund individual who was rather gruff and opinionated in his demeanor. In spite of all the lung cancer patients that he had operated on over his long and illustrious career, he continued to smoke cigarettes, justifying it by saying that the only ones who got cancer were the ones who quit smoking. When I was his student, Dr. Gale was nearing the end of his career, and most of his surgeries were carried out by his senior residents under his supervision. He often entered the operating suite after the chest was open and rib resections for exposure were complete. He would then begin his part of the operation, isolating the tumor or the lobes to be resected, ligating major blood vessels, and closing major bronchi. At times, the entire procedure was carried out by the senior resident while Dr. Gale observed. After the procedure Dr. Gale would leave the operating room to have a cigarette. He had a superb senior surgery resident, Dr. Bill Kisken, who was very knowledgeable and possessed great surgical hands. The intern on the service was a woman and, unfortunately for her, Dr. Gale was not a great believer in female doctors. With this disadvantage, she proceeded to make several critical mistakes on her first day on the service. At the surgical suite she began to scrub her hands, as we all did for at least 10 minutes, but committed the grievous sin of using Dr. Gale's "private" sink. When Dr. Gale arrived he quickly told her to go elsewhere and scrub. The case began with her as the second assistant to Dr. Gale and Dr. Kisken. She sinned again by calling suture, "string". Dr. Gale was seething behind his mask, but, under reasonable control, suggested that she go to the surgery ward and make rounds on the patients and he would join her later. He never let her return to the operating room, which was to my advantage, because I moved up to second assistant. Whenever Dr. Gale took a cigarette break, Dr. Kisken took over and I became first assistant. This allowed me to get my gloved hands into the operating field and hold retractors, sponges, and hemostats. I can't think of another medical school experience where I had so much fun and was so excited.

The Department of Medicine was chaired by Dr. Ovid Meyer, who always had a red rose pinned to the lapel of his white lab coat. He was a stickler for detail and always walked through the doorway onto the medical ward at exactly 8 a.m.. On one occasion while making rounds at a patient's bedside he asked me to present the case to the residents and other medical students. Knowing his fastidious nature, I began a very thorough and accurate recitation. He finally cut me off and said he had never met such a talkative Norwegian in his life, which embarrassed me and drew chuckles from the patient as well as the resident and intern on the service.

On a different medical ward we had a staff doctor whom we soon found out was totally incompetent and, I think, slightly insane. During a teaching session at his gastroenterology laboratory, he had one of my female classmates sit on his lap while he expounded about some medical condition. His bizarre, if not totally inappropriate quirks, were not as alarming as his judgment, however. He was so erratic, in fact, that we were concerned for the well-being of our patients. For instance, he would inexplicably order the resident physician to discontinue insulin on diabetic patients. I don't know if this staff doctor ever noticed, but whenever he was on the ward, the most seriously-ill patients were spirited away to the laboratory or X-ray departments for "testing". We even temporarily hid some patients in the bathrooms! It was rumored that this doctor was kept on staff because he had served as the private physician for numerous state legislators and, therefore, was a useful lobbying tool for the medical school to obtain funds from the state. I don't know if this was true, but I began to suspect that this guy was not the only off-kilter doctor allowed to practice medicine. It was a strange realization for me to accept.

On the opposite end of the spectrum, was the doctor who served as my preceptor (a physician that senior students were assigned to for a period of three to four months). There were preceptorships in Monroe, La Crosse, Eau Claire, Marshfield, Milwaukee, Wausau, and even in small town Viroqua. I was sent to Wausau to work with the hospital Chief-of-Staff Dr. Merritt L. Jones, who had a surgery and orthopedic service along with his associate Dr. Roy Larson. Dr. Jones was elderly but very sharp mentally, and a sage who reminded me of a benevolent great uncle. My time with him gave me an excellent chance to closely observe an office practice as well as a hospital practice. I watched him as he smoothly deflected political machinations from jealous rivals, (something I didn't realize existed) and as he expertly assessed disability and Workmen's Compensation examinations, which required him to testify in court (another aspect of medicine I hadn't known about). When Dr. Jones was not in surgery he saw patients in his office, sometimes determining that the problem was psychophysiologic (physical symptoms or illness caused by emotional or behavioral problems). He then would turn to me and say, "Lowell, go in the back and get me some of those pink pills," which he prescribed to the patient. The pills were aspirin tablets. Thus, I saw that the art of medicine might at times involve artifice (subtle deception and ingenuity) and yet still result in effective and responsible care.

It was incredibly instructive to passively observe experienced doctors, both good and bad. Sometimes the lessons I learned occurred well after the educational moment passed. One evening I was called to the delivery room for a lady who was moving rapidly through labor and I realized that the attending doctor was not present. Because I had good OB training as a student in Madison I felt confident that I could deliver the baby, but just as the baby was "crowning" and ready to pop out of the vaginal canal, the attending doctor arrived, so I stepped aside to watch. To my amazement the doctor pushed the baby's head back in the delivery canal and then put forceps on the head before proceeding to deliver the child. I could not believe what I had just seen. I learned later that the medical fee for a forceps delivery was higher than for a simple vaginal delivery. At that moment I was simply standing in muted shock. Unfortunately, it wouldn't be the last time.

On another occasion I was asked to come to a medical ward of the hospital and start an intravenous fluid line on a postoperative female patient because the attending doctor was busy seeing patients in his office. When I arrived to start the IV, the young woman had very low blood pressure and was, in fact, near total vascular collapse (shock) and barely conscious. I made numerous attempts to get a needle into the vein but was unsuccessful. I asked her some questions but she was too obtunded to give me any meaningful answers. When I reviewed her medical records, I found that the patient had previously had tuberculosis. I made a diagnosis that the tuberculosis had destroyed her adrenal glands and that she was suffering from Addison's disease (an inability to produce the adrenal catecholamines, such as epinephrine and nor-epinephrine, which are necessary to support blood pressure). As a student fearful of overstepping my bounds, I had the nurses call the attending physician to explain the situation to him and to request that he come to see the patient. He either did not agree with my diagnosis or the gravity of the situation, and did not come to see the patient until after his office hours—but he was there when she died. I was mortified at the time and even more so at the next general medical staff meeting when a review of all deaths in the hospital were discussed. After a short discussion, it was decided that this patient's death was not preventable. Again, I remained in shocked silence feeling strangely outraged and complicit at the same time. I berate myself for not calling the attending doctor directly and boldly asserting my belief that the patient would die unless she was promptly attended to. As a lowly medical student, my courage failed me, and I carry the guilt of that day with me to the present.

As terrifying as it was to be forced into situations of making critical decisions without another doctor present, these moments could also serve as proof that I could face the situation rationally, use proper judgement, and act on the issue under consideration. I will try to counter these bad experiences by relating one of the finest experiences of my preceptorship and an experience that I find gratifying to this day.

I was asked to see a patient very late in the evening after I had assisted on his surgery earlier in the day. He had lung cancer and the surgery was difficult, prolonged, and maybe inadvisable. There were no CT scans in those days to assess the extent of the tumor and it was well accepted that surgery with the removal of as much tumor as possible was highly justified. Unfortunately, the lung tumor was adherent from its left upper lobe location to surrounding structures including the aorta, the main blood vessel coming from the heart. After a long and tedious attempt to remove the bulk of the tumor, the chest was closed with very little hope for the patient's survival. That evening, close to midnight, I was requested to come to the patient's room to place a Foley catheter in his bladder as he was unable to pass his urine. A young nurse, Shirley Manicke, who recently graduated from nursing school in Eau Claire, was assigned as his special nurse for the night. She assisted me in my attempts to care for the patient and to place the catheter. I was unsuccessful in passing the catheter past his prostate gland. He was obviously miserable from the bladder expansion, and by examination his bladder extended up above his umbilicus. Attempts were made to reach the attending surgeon but he was unavailable. I then requested a pediatric feeding tube which was smaller but stiffer than the

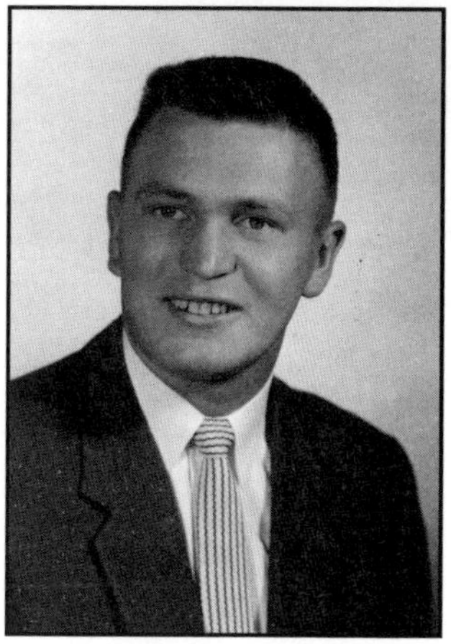

My graduation photo

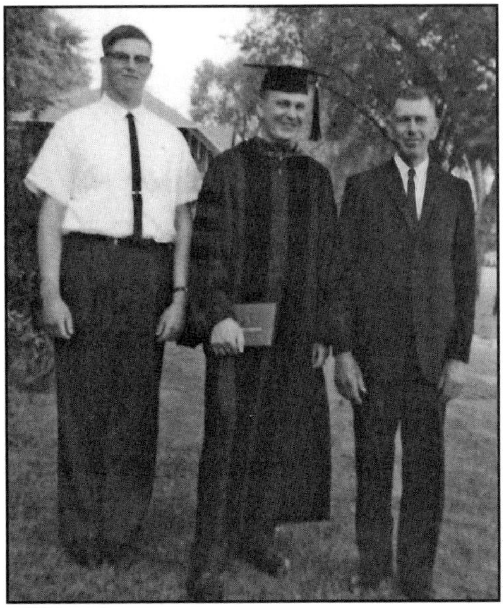

Medical School graduation day with brother, Gordy, and Dad

Foley catheter. I was able to pass this through the prostate into the bladder. As the bladder slowly drained the patient became much more comfortable. The young nurse, Shirley, remained with the patient throughout the night. I was very impressed with her sincere concern and skill in attending and calming the patient. In the morning when the attending doctor arrived and heard the story of the nighttime adventure, he was upset at my brazen behavior because it was not standard medical care. I probably should have consulted a urologist to place the Foley catheter using filaform guides or place a suprapubic catheter tube directly through the abdominal wall into the bladder. In spite of his scolding, I felt gratified that I was able to solve the problem by improvising. The patient was very thankful. I also feel fortunate that this wonderful young nurse, with her kind words, gave me encouragement to try to do what was best for the patient.

It was during my junior and senior years that the dean of the medical school, Dr. John Z. Bowers came into direct conflict with numerous staff physicians especially in the department of surgery. Dr. Bowers envisioned the creation of very strong services in various departments and the creation of a medical school that was of equal esteem with the best medical schools in the country. In his rather unbending dictatorial manner he brought in top-notch chiefs of service in many departments who in turn recruited other highly-talented individuals to increase the prestige and medical expertise of their departments. He was successful in doing so in the department of pediatrics, obstetrics, and neurology. As a result, some of the least qualified and older physicians were forced out. He then attempted to bring in a new chief of surgery without consulting the members of the surgery department, ENT, urology, ophthalmology, and orthopedics. The personnel and leaders of these departments along with many in the department of medicine saw the handwriting on the wall for their fiefdoms and conspired to block his nomination. They insisted that the new chief of surgery should come from within the department of general surgery, specifically choosing Dr. Anthony Curreri, a prestigious surgeon. After a rather long and heated battle with much media coverage and government legislative interference, Dr. Bowers withdrew his nomination for the new chief of surgery and he himself resigned. This was a very sad day for the residents, interns, and medical students who were very supportive of Dr. Bowers. We realized that the people he had brought in were responsible for the best teaching we experienced.

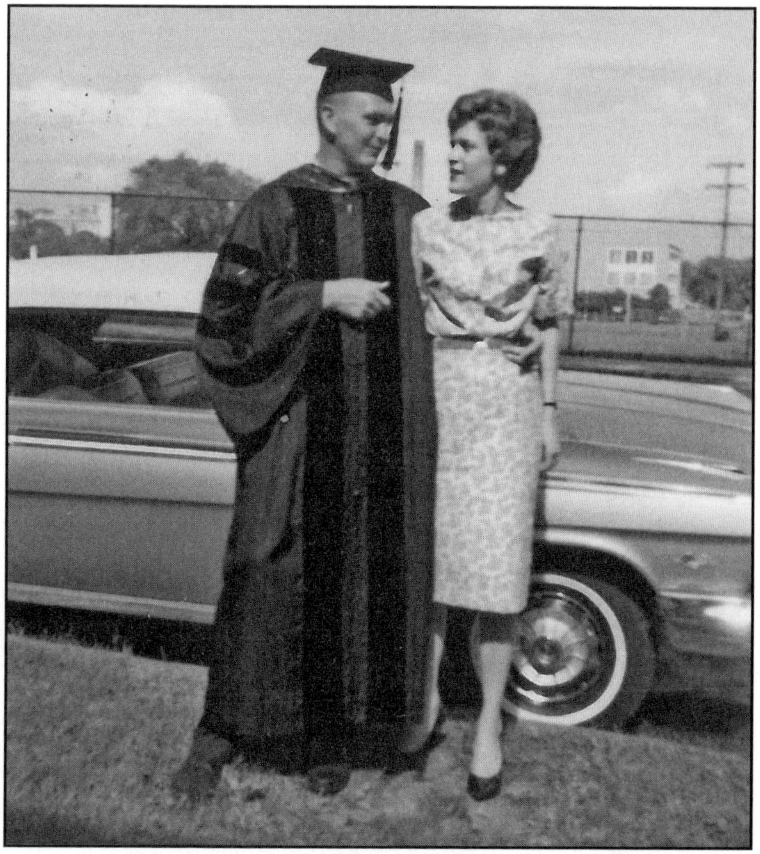

My fiancee, Mary, and me, on graduation day, 1962

By the time I graduated from medical school in the spring of 1962, I felt I was prepared to move on to the next phase of my training. I was very happy on the day I received my diploma from the University of Wisconsin designating me as fulfilling the requirements for the degree of Doctor of Medicine. I walked across the stage of the fieldhouse to receive my diploma escorted by a staff doctor, Dr. William Kieckhofer, of the Obstetrics and Gynecology department. In the audience, I was very proud to have as my guests, my dad, my high school principal, A. O. Lee, and my newly engaged bride-to-be, Mary Dressendorfer. At this point I felt as if the world lay at my doorstep.

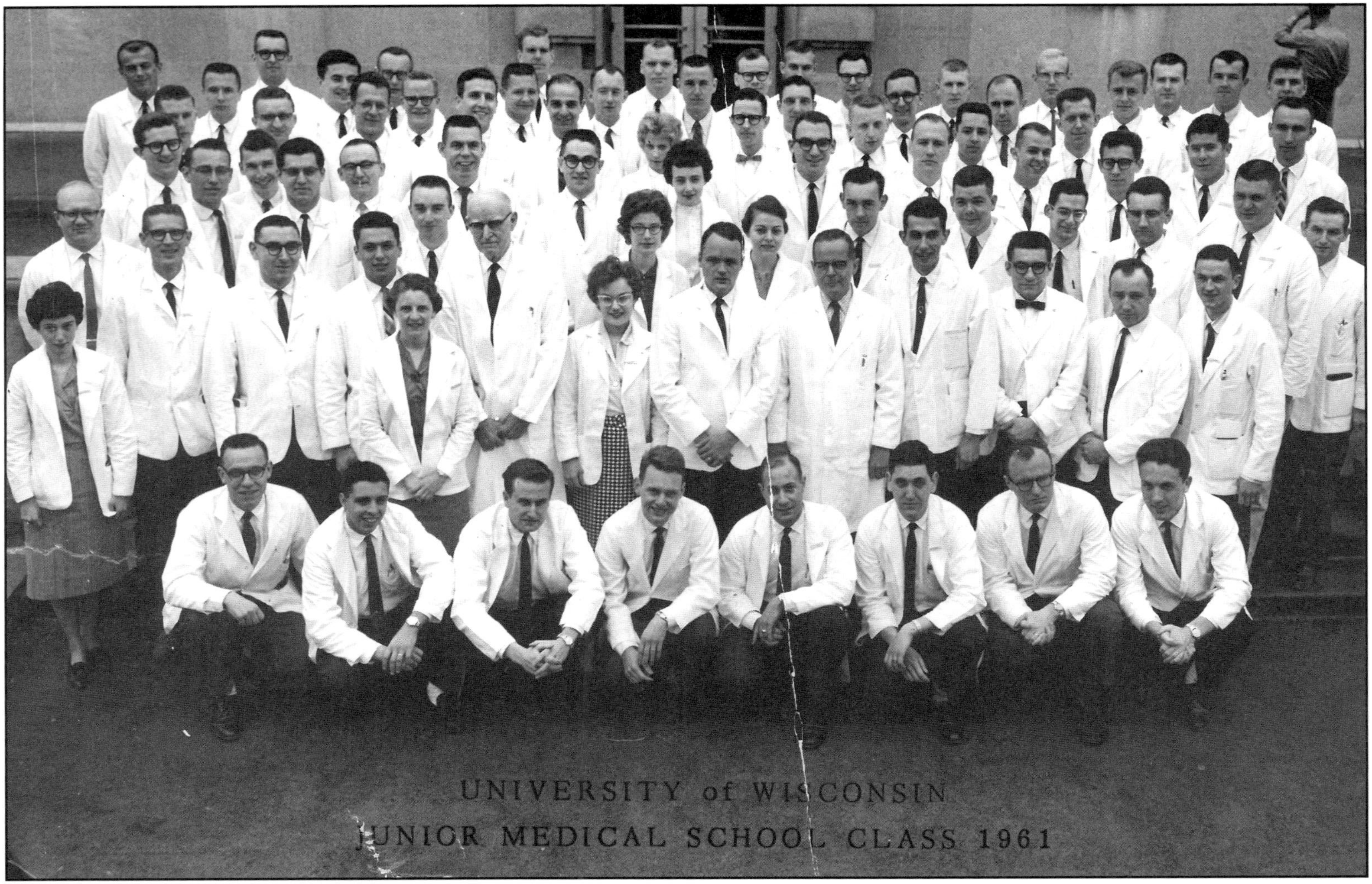

Dr. Schmidt, Chief of Surgery, standing sixth from left, and Dean Bowers, fifth from right. I am second from right in the third row

Chapter Seven

INTERNSHIP

(1962-1963)

With the pomp and circumstance of graduation fading from memory and the ink on my medical diploma barely dry, I embarked on the next phase of my medical education—internship. Senior medical students apply to internship programs throughout the country and the hospitals rate the applicants to match the candidates to the slots available. When it was all said and done, I was accepted at Milwaukee Lutheran Hospital in Milwaukee, Wisconsin, a very reputable general hospital with strong programs in surgery, medicine, and obstetrics-gynecology. Since I was unsure of my career direction, I chose to rotate through different specialties. Each one—surgery, pediatrics, OB/GYN, internal medicine—would last three months.

> *The American Medical Association*
>
> *extends congratulations to you*
>
> *upon the occasion of your graduation*
>
> *from Medical School*
>
> *and welcomes you to*
>
> *The Medical Profession*

There were nine interns at Milwaukee Lutheran in 1962-1963. The hospital also had a residency program training surgical residents, OB/GYN residents, and medical residents, and therefore, the entire house-staff consisted of about 20 young physicians in training.

The surgery rotation inaugurated my intern experience and on my very first day I was assigned to assist a plastic surgeon performing a facelift operation. This, like most plastic surgery procedures, was very tedious and consumed several hours. The incision extended from ear to ear, following just below the jaw line where the excess sagging tissue was removed. The incisional repair involved placement of scores of tiny hair-thin sutures very close together. Unfortunately for me, there was not much for an assistant to do in a case like this except watch the technique of the surgeon. I don't remember being bored but it was rather monotonous to stand there attentively for hours on end. Following the surgery, I finished my other duties of the day, taking histories and performing physical examinations on patients who were scheduled for surgery the following day. That night when I was the intern on-call for surgery, I received a call at about 11 p.m. that the patient who had received the facelift was being taken back to surgery. The area under the surgical flap became very swollen due to a large hematoma (blood clot) that now required evacuation and re-repair. Once again I stood at the surgeon's side as he removed each carefully sewn suture, coagulated the bleeding sites, irrigated the wound with saline solution, and, eventually, replaced each stitch one by one. After what seemed like an eternity staring at this patient's jaw line, the procedure finally ended in the early morning and I prepared for the full day's work ahead of me as an assistant to other surgeons. Needless to say, I was exhausted. But I was lucid enough to realize that I didn't want to enter the field of plastic surgery.

Overall the surgery rotation was very pleasant and instructive, and I discovered in the operating room (OR) that most surgical procedures are fairly unvarying—an appendectomy is an appendectomy—but, the surgeons' personalities and preferences made each day different. It was quickly apparent that surgeons carried a lot of ego into the OR, which is somewhat understandable as they are the ones responsible for what happens on the operating table. I also observed that this extra self-confidence fostered some professional jealousies and petty grudges. One very skilled and speedy surgeon would often complete his surgery and then enter other operating rooms and chide the surgeons operating there, asking why they were taking so long. He also liked to brag about patients who had gone to Houston to have their aortic aneurysms repaired by the world famous Dr. Michael DeBakey only to find that they would have to have the proccdure redone by him. Exactly how many times this happened, I have no idea, but the retelling of the story numbered well over twenty.

Another surgeon I assisted was very fussy, insisting that he always operate in a "dry field" (suture-ligating or cauterizing every tiny bleeder). He also believed in teaching the surgery residents and interns to observe his compulsive technique, but he rarely allowed any of us to become directly involved. On one occasion he, rather surprisingly, did ask the surgery resident if he would like to perform part of the operation, to which the resident replied sarcastically, "It would be my distinct pleasure!" Although we were annoyed by his fastidious nature, we always felt that the quality of the surgeon's work was outstanding and instructive.

As time went on I felt I was getting a grip on what it meant to be a surgeon and how sometimes your results were only as good as the cooperation and health of your patient. There was a senior and highly-respected surgeon whom I assisted in performing a cholecystectomy (gallbladder removal). The female patient was rather obese and, therefore, the surgery was difficult. I remember the doctor working his way through the layers of fat on the abdominal wall, and, as he nervously shifted his weight from foot to foot, he became more frustrated, commenting disgustedly, "Nothing but goose grease!" The following day, while we made our surgical rounds on the ward, the patient—apparently a very prominent lady in the community—begged the doctor to allow her to leave the hospital so that she could attend a social function that evening. The surgeon strongly discouraged her request but finally gave in and allowed her to go on pass for a few hours. As might be expected, the woman dehisced (separated and disrupted) her wound with multiple sutures in the skin and fatty tissues pulling loose. She was returned to surgery in the middle of the night for a repeat repair of the wound. Needless to say, the surgeon was livid (at his patient and, no doubt, himself), and he vowed he would never give in to such a request again.

I was learning that speaking with patients on any given day could be educational, heartwarming, depressing, or exhausting. On one occasion I found the interaction to be personally helpful. A "playboy" patient was admitted to our hospital with acute abdominal pain related to peritonitis from a ruptured hole in his intestine that required surgery. While on a recent Caribbean island excursion he developed acute appendicitis and had his appendix removed. Just before returning to Milwaukee he went sailing and was thrown against the shipboard railing by waves in a rough sea. When he arrived at our hospital he was acutely ill. Surgery revealed he had "blown out" the sutured stump where the appendix was removed, allowing bowel contents to enter the abdominal-peritoneal cavity. The re-repair was successful, but he spent an extended period of time in the hospital with drainage tubes in his abdomen while receiving antibiotics. As I got to know him during my daily rounds, I started asking him about the Caribbean islands and told him that my fiancé and I were considering a Caribbean honeymoon. He sent me with a personal recommendation to his travel agent and suggested that we go to Jamaica and stay at the Half Moon Resort, and that is exactly what we did. He did not mention that a September wedding meant we would be going to Jamaica during the hurricane season. With our dumb luck, however, the weather was wonderful.

After the surgery rotation I moved to the medicine service, which exposed me to multiple internal medicine specialists (Internists); a few had subspecialty training, which was uncommon in those days. My role as an intern on this service consisted of taking patient histories, conducting physical exams, and making rounds on these patients with the attending physicians. I really did not get to manage patient care. When I wrote orders on the chart I had to have them co-signed by the attending physician. One internist, who re-combed his hair before entering every patient's room, asked me to hand him the chart at the bedside as if I were a pageboy presenting the chart on a silken pillow. He recognized my disinterest with this pompous arrangement that was non-educational, and said, "Lowell, I don't think you like making rounds with me." I assured him I was pleased to work with and observe him, as I put tongue-in-cheek and replaced my pout with a smile.

During this rotation, I was required to take night-call on a regular basis which meant working a 36-hour shift, sometimes with sleep and sometimes without. On one occasion I went to sleep in the intern-resident quarters after a very tiring day and later was called by the nurses to come down to attend a patient who was not doing very well. At least, that's what I was later told. Apparently still asleep, I hung up the phone. The nurse called me again a bit later and asked if I was going to come to see the patient and, still sleep-talking, I responded by saying, "No". Fortunately for the patient, the nurse was able to contact the medical resident who responded promptly. The next morning I was accosted by the attending physician, the medical resident, and nurses, all of whom were asking why I did not respond in an appropriate fashion during the night. I sheepishly explained that I had absolutely no recollection of the phone calls or of any conversations. I was totally embarrassed, but more importantly, I was scared. I realized that I could easily lose my internship appointment. Fortunately, the medical resident, Dr. John Brown, put in a good word for me, and between us we were able to satisfy the physician and nursing staff. From that time forward, I always placed the telephone well away from the bedside so that I had to get out of bed to answer any calls. This tactic seemed to work, and even many years later in private practice I insisted on putting the telephone on my wife's side of the bed so at least if I started to drift back to sleep, she would be awake (and annoyed) enough to give me a sharp jab in the ribs.

I remember visiting an elderly Jewish lady on medical rounds. I inquired how she was doing and if there was anything I could do for her. Each day I got the same answer: "Dr. Petermann, just give me my Metamucils (stool softeners) and I'll be all right." She never did get my name right and was totally oblivious to anything else that I was saying. One of the internists explained this phenomenon by noting that, "You know you are getting old if the only thing you worry about are your bowels."

The cases I saw as an intern were mostly routine, but sometimes they could present unique conditions. I remember the odd case of a man who entered the hospital because of severe and unrelenting pain in his right foot. He was a salesman who managed a children's shoe store that had an X-ray machine to check his patron's shoe sizes and fit. This wasn't unusual at the time, although it is illegal now. He would put his foot in the X-ray machine and fluoroscope it along with the child's foot. The discrepancy in the size of his and the child's foot bones was hilarious for his patrons to see and the man was usually guaranteed a sale. Unfortunately, the continual exposure to radiation resulted in necrosis and destruction of skin and soft tissue structures of his right foot and ankle such that the bones and tendons were clearly visible. There was no question that he had to have his lower leg amputated, which he did. It was a painful irony for this shoe salesman, I'm sure, to suffer a phenomenon called "phantom limb", (a sensation that the amputated limb was still present). He remained with physical discomfort for the rest of his life. This was one of the first of countless instances where I saw how we could "solve" a patient's medical problem, but not necessarily make him better.

In another case, a young girl in her teens was admitted to the hospital after a grand-mal epileptic seizure. Extensive neurologic evaluation revealed that she had a loud bruit, or "whooshing" noise, audible with a stethoscope, over her right eyeball and at her right temple. It is the only time I have ever experienced this phenomena although I have often ruled it out as part of my examination of any patient with a neurologic problem. A subsequent arteriogram showed a large arterial-venous malformation of the brain behind her right eye. This is a congenital abnormality where arteries and veins are connected directly in a convoluted hodgepodge, not through the normal capillary networks. It was considered inoperable. Modern techniques might involve selective embolization of small foreign bodies like small BBs into the vascular structure to stimulate clot formation and avoid increase in size or rupture of the malformation. This case was another initiation into what is possible in medicine and what is impossible. I felt a degrading sense of impotence as our medical team had to tell the patient and her family the diagnosis and inform them that the only thing we could do for her was prescribe anti-seizure medications. Her prognosis was morbid, probably mortal, and certainly unfortunate.

Some of my happier moments of the year were thanks to Dr. Bruce Brewer, an orthopedic surgeon, the team doctor for the Milwaukee Braves (the renamed Milwaukee Brewers came to the city from Seattle several years after the Braves were spirited away to Atlanta). I loved baseball and if I was not tied up doing something else, I would make a point of seeing if I could work with Dr. Brewer, which resulted in some lucky encounters with my favorite team's players. I assisted Dr. Brewer in injecting cortisone into many pitchers' shoulders and elbows—and, amazingly, into the right shoulder joint of third baseman Eddie Mathews, a superstar who hit more than 500 home runs in his career. Dr. Brewer reminded me that although this was very exciting and heady stuff for me, working on arms of players that were being paid exorbitant amounts of money to perform in their profession was not to be taken lightly. I nodded, gravely, but I never got over the giddy feeling of coming in contact with real major leaguers. And despite Dr. Brewers' admonitions, many of my interactions with the players made me smile. I had one patient, for example, who entered the hospital with a painful boil in his armpit. The evaluation and treatment was rather straightforward, and I always looked forward to my conversations with him when I would visit him on rounds every morning. Once, when I was looking at his chart, I glanced at the admission data at the top, which included his name, date of birth, insurance, etc. One blank requested to know his occupation. He did not respond by saying he was a professional baseball player or a member of the Milwaukee Braves. He just wrote, "Right Fielder".

The best part of the relationship to the Milwaukee Braves in 1962-63 was that our hospital had two free passes to all the home games so a physician was in attendance in case any injury might occur to a player. The hospital's box seats were right behind home plate with a great view of the entire stadium. Because my wife and I were both avid baseball fans, we requested the tickets whenever I was not working. Because the other doctors were not as interested, we were able to utilize the tickets frequently. While attending one Sunday afternoon game with my wife, a clubhouse attendant came to our seats and requested that I follow him. I was taken into the visiting team locker room and out into the dugout during the game. The Braves were playing Philadelphia and the Phillies third baseman, Don Hoak, had just jammed his thumb while diving for a ground ball, but he refused to go to the locker room. It was a bad sprain and I advised him to apply ice and to get X-rays after the game. While I was in the dugout the word spread that a doctor was there and soon I was holding sick call for several other players, including the center fielder who had a sore throat. I have to admit that, opposing team or not, having an excuse to stay in the dugout and see the game from their vantage point was an amazing indulgence. Overhearing the player chatter, I heard, "We're gonna get to this guy," meaning the Braves pitcher. I agreed, as it was obvious that the pitcher had lost some velocity on his fastball by this stage of the game. A little later I was there when the manager of the Phillies, Gene Mauch, sent Frank Torre (Joe's brother), up to pinch-hit during the rally that followed. Finally, it was clear that I had no more patients to see and that it was time to rejoin the general public in the stands. When I returned, my wife looked exasperated, saying, "Where have you been all this time?" When I replied, "I was in the dugout," she did not believe me.

Although there would be no baseball players passing through the OB/GYN ward, I was nevertheless really looking forward to my three-month rotation there. I had a good experience during my OB rotation in medical school and I figured that my internship would simply cement this as my future career path. Soon after starting my OB rotation, however, it became apparent to me that nothing was set in stone. The internship obstetrics experience of delivering babies day in and day out and night in and night out left me physically tired and always in a recovery mode. Mentally, it was no longer a challenge to me to assist deliveries and perform episiotomy repairs. Scrubbing in for GYN surgery and holding retractors for hysterectomies became so routine that I felt that, even as an intern, I could do them in my sleep. Perhaps more critical, however, was the idealistic disenchantment I felt with certain members of the OB/GYN staff who routinely induced their patient's deliveries with intravenous Pitocin or scheduled caesarean section deliveries on Fridays so that the doctor would have his weekend free. Although it was disappointing to remain without a clear career path, at least I was content with my decision to keep searching.

The pediatrics rotation at Children's Hospital was another learning experience that taught me what I would not want to do for the rest of my career. Moreover, by ruling out pediatrics I was also ruling out general practice, because pediatrics and OB/GYN are a big part of general practice. To this day, I hate seeing sick kids and feel ill-equipped to provide care and comfort, whether they are patients, my children, my grandchildren, or the children of friends or neighbors. It is just so unfair for these innocent, young, trusting individuals to deal with an illness, or worse, a malignancy. While at Children's Hospital I worked under the supervision of the pediatric residency physicians who were very helpful in teaching the interns and medical students, but it was also apparent that these residents were overworked and always tired from being on night-call with no sleep. Having to do venipunctures to draw blood samples from babies and small children or try to start intravenous needles and catheters for the administration of fluids and antibiotics was no easy task for any of us. The best veins to be utilized for this purpose were on the scalp and the child would usually have to be restrained by strapping them to a board so that the procedure could be completed. Although this seems like torture, the justification was that what we were doing was diagnostic, therapeutic, and carried out to improve their situation.

I remember, vividly, a young child, probably about six years old, who was admitted with a very high fever of better than 105°. Examination revealed a severe tonsillitis and strep throat but even worse was the presence of a paratonsillar abscess that was almost occluding the upper pharyngeal airway. In addition to the IV fluids, antibiotics, and fever control measures including an ice bath, it was obvious that the patient needed to go to surgery to lance the abscess, drain it, and clear the airway. Meanwhile, the father of the child kept on insisting that his kid's illness was not very serious and that we should just give him a shot of penicillin and send him home. This was not a case of parental denial. It was clear that this guy was just a jerk and it made me so angry that I wanted to pin him against the wall. Instead, the tactful approach of the pediatric resident, Dr. Montgomery, finally convinced the father to consent to his son's surgery. Then, he promptly left to go home, seeming not to care what the end result might be. It was heartbreaking and dumbfounding. But, I had learned from this encounter that a cool head and tactfulness were superior to argumentation and anger.

On September 8, 1962, three months into my internship, I was married to Mary Ruth Dressendorfer in Marshfield, Wisconsin. During that first year we had very little time together, due to my hectic schedule, and we survived on $50 a month for groceries and gas. Once a week, however, we did treat ourselves by going to Dimicelli's, a neighborhood bar, for their large hamburgers and a couple of beers.

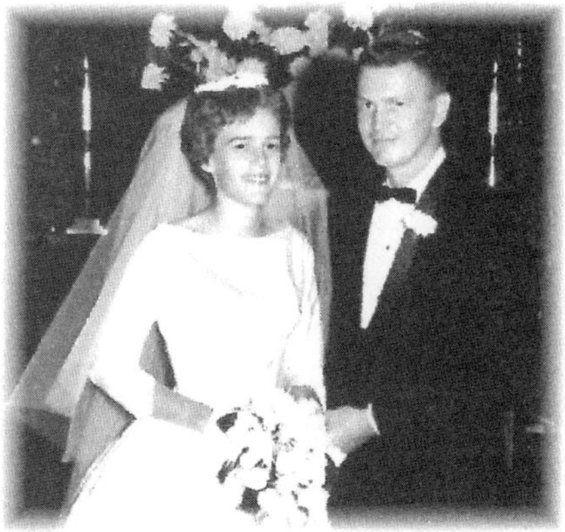

September 8, 1962

When I was not on-call for a weekend, my wife and I often drove north to our hometowns for some relaxation. We would also scavenger several pounds of butter and a bushel of potatoes from my dad and brother on our family farm. If I could not get off for a weekend I might ask my good friend Wayne Simonson and his new wife, Ginny, who were also working in Milwaukee, to bring back some fresh produce for me. We had both been married within a month of each other and had been attendants in each other's wedding.

One weekend when the Simonson's were heading north after dark, in a rainstorm, a car turned directly in front of them on Highway 100 as they crossed Capitol Drive resulting in a catastrophic accident. Wayne and Ginny were rushed to Milwaukee County General Hospital and given superior care. Ginny survived but Wayne's injuries were mortal. The hospital did not have any emergency information for next of kin. The only thing they found in his billfold was a telephone number and the name "Pete" on the slip of paper. Wayne had kept this so he could contact me when he returned from his trip home. When the County Hospital staff dialed this number they were surprised to find that it was

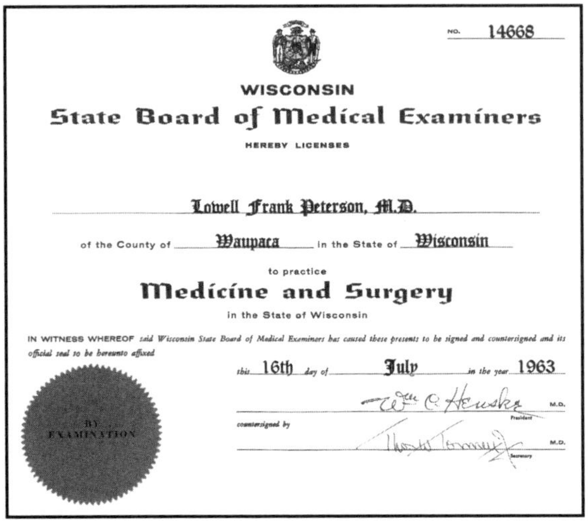
NO. 14668

WISCONSIN
State Board of Medical Examiners
HEREBY LICENSES

Lowell Frank Peterson, M.D.

of the County of Waupaca in the State of Wisconsin

to practice
Medicine and Surgery
in the State of Wisconsin

IN WITNESS WHEREOF said Wisconsin State Board of Medical Examiners has caused these presents to be signed and countersigned and its official seal to be hereunto affixed

this 16th day of July in the year 1963

M.D. President

countersigned by

M.D. Secretary

BY EXAMINATION

a phone number of another hospital. The telephone operator at my hospital did not make the connection between the name on the piece of paper and me. Through further investigation Wayne's parents were finally notified and I was made aware of the situation the following day. Mary and I visited the county hospital and were shocked beyond belief. Nothing in my past medical experience had prepared me for what I saw before me. Motionless, dependent on life support, bruised and battered, my friend lay in front of me, brain dead. The resident physician briefed me on the hopeless situation. I met with his parents but was basically speechless and incapable of expressing any meaningful comfort to them as they awaited the loss of their only child. That afternoon I went back to our small apartment, threw myself on the bed, and cried like a baby. I was losing one of my best friends. Several days later I would serve as a pallbearer for Wayne at his funeral, delivering his flag-draped casket to its final resting place.

Incredibly, I found that time kept moving forward and I returned to my daily chores as an intern. The shock stayed with me for some time. I believe that I learned from this experience as I went on to deal with seriously ill and injured patients in the future. I tried to keep my emotions in check, separating myself from the patient lying in the hospital bed, so that I could continue to treat them with empathy without losing my focus. But, after Wayne's passing I found that I could no longer banish thoughts of family and friends that the person was leaving behind. In my career, patient care and social responsibility to their loved ones, has never been impersonal. It is the Christian way. It is The Golden Rule.

Chapter Eight

AIR FORCE MEDICINE

(1963-1966)

In 1988 we took our children on a nostalgic trip to Okinawa, 25 years after arriving there for the first time. As we approached the island by air, the familiar topography became readily apparent and the memories and emotions of a momentous experience began to surface. Kitty said, "Dad, aren't you excited?" I was so wrapped up in my emotions that I could not respond—but she knew. Memories of the camaraderie with my fellow physicians and the pilots, the Kadena Dispensary experience, the deployments to Southeast Asia, and the flights all over the Far East were racing through my head. Watching the modern fighter jets launch from Kadena Air Base and visiting the houses where we lived was also nostalgic. Yes, Kitty, I only partially controlled the tears of joy associated with this reminiscence.

♥

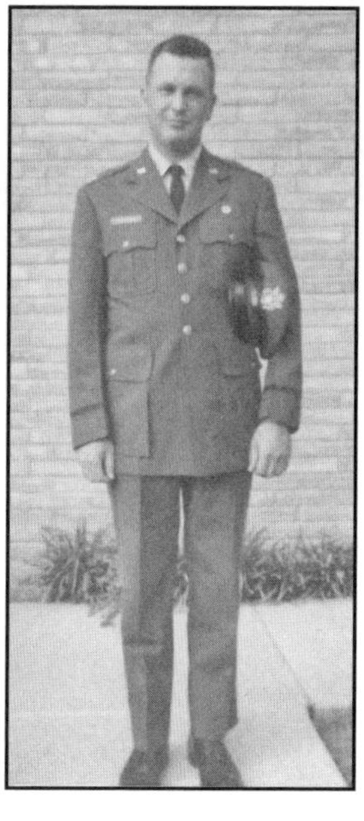

In July of 1963 at the request of the United States government, I reported to flight surgeon's school at Brooks Air Force Base in San Antonio, Texas. I spent twelve weeks there before being deployed to my permanent duty assignment at Kadena Air Force Base in Okinawa, Japan. The course of study included lectures explaining air force protocol and regulations, medical qualification and disqualification for flying status, aircraft accident investigation, and, of course, how to fill out the myriad of forms required by military bureaucracy. Practical experience in decompression chambers, ejection seat trainers, jumping from parachute landing practice towers, and, escaping parachutes while being dragged across the Texas turf with a tractor were meant to prepare me for worst-case scenarios. A back seat ride in a T-33 jet made the school experience all worthwhile. The pilot even let me fly the airplane for part of the flight and instructed me how to read the instruments and make aileron rolls.

Soon after arriving at Kadena, I began work in the medical dispensary. The colonel in command was likely a stellar physician in his heyday but when I knew him he was at the end of his career and a bit senile. At this point in his career he was mostly concerned with following protocol or filling out paperwork, and certainly discouraging flight surgeons from doing anything but work in the clinic. Fortunately, he was soon given a proper retirement party and we said, “sayonara”. The new and subsequent commanders made my job easier and more interesting. They realized how important it was for flight surgeons to get to know the pilots and their families personally before any of them required medical services at the dispensary. This meant that I got to spend much more time on the flight-line with my assigned squadron members and not just see them for their annual physical exam.

I was assigned to the 12th TAC fighter squadron of the 18th tactical fighter wing. The 18th was made up of three squadrons flying F-105 single engine jet fighter-bombers—the 12th, the 44th, and the 67th—and a fourth squadron, the 15th, flying RF-101 reconnaissance jets. I was very fortunate to be accepted as their “Doc” by these skilled “jet jockeys”. The camaraderie was especially strengthened in combat during our squadron deployment to Korat, Thailand, in Southeast Asia, during the Vietnam air war. The war also strengthened the commitment of our medical commanders to the flight surgeon’s mission. The 105s and their pilots were targeted on a daily basis by anti-aircraft artillery, small arms fire, and later by surface-to-air (SAM) missiles and MiG fighter-interceptors furnished by the Russians. The safe return from a mission was not guaranteed and, indeed, some pilots I knew did not come back. Those who survived lived with constant psychological stress, whether it was openly acknowledged or not. The possibility of taking a direct missile hit, or of being shot down, captured, and tortured by the enemy was a constant threat. It was no surprise to me that the pilots welcomed the relaxing atmosphere of the bar at the officer’s club every evening. I realized that my job as the pilots’ physician should extend beyond doling out anti-malaria pills, aspirin, antacids, or filling out forms. I needed to be there—in the squadron briefing rooms for pre- and post-flight discourse, at operations headquarters to understand their missions, and at the officer’s club—to know what these men were assigned to do and how they coped with doing it. Offering whatever psychological support I could was more important than anything else I did.

When I was back at Kadena, I was required to work in the general medical dispensary as well as in the flight surgeon's office on a regular basis and to take night- and weekend-call as the Medical Officer of the Day (M.O.D.). In the military, free access to medical care for service personnel and families was considered a right, as well as a privilege and, therefore, we, as medical service providers, were obliged to evaluate and treat all comers. There were about 15 doctors at the dispensary who were general medical officers, along with five or six flight surgeons. We would see patients from 7:30 a.m. until 4:30 p.m. except for a 15-minute coffee break in the morning and a 30-minute break for lunch. A patient was allotted ten minutes for a visit, in which time the doctor would obtain a history of the chief complaint, complete a physical examination, order appropriate lab work or X-rays, write any necessary prescriptions, and explain as thoroughly as possible the diagnosis and recommended course of action. I found that I could accomplish this in the short time allowed and that it was an excellent learning experience. This format sharpened my observational skills so that within seconds of the patient entering my office, I could determine how ill they were without ever asking a question.

Many of the office visits, in fact, were medically unnecessary, but by simply reassuring the patient that all-was-well, their anxiety was relieved. At times, the open-access system also fostered a kind of "come and get it" mentality, where families descended on the dispensary in hopes of stocking up on supplies. On Sunday evenings in particular, the M.O.D. would not be busy and almost bored until 9 p.m. when the TV program, "Gunsmoke", ended. Then the floodgates would open and the dependents (wives and children) along with their servicemen husbands would descend to receive their free medical care. I couldn't really blame them. They knew that the servicemen would be going back to work on Monday morning at their duty stations, leaving their wives to deal with any family medical problems. Usually, the onslaught would be over by midnight or 1 a.m. and the

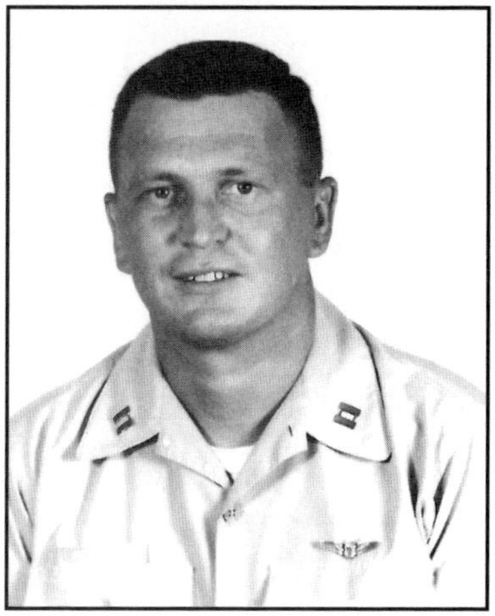

M.O.D. could get some sleep and leave any routine medical care during the night to the corpsman on duty. I don't mean to belittle the medical needs of the patients who came to the dispensary during usual business hours because most of them did have legitimate medical complaints. It was always very interesting to see the wives of newly promoted sergeants who had been advanced to noncommissioned officer status or wives of those newly promoted to Lieutenant Colonel. These wives would often be very demanding of what they felt should be done for them or their children, (i.e. Penicillin for the common cold). When I would advise something different than what they wanted, the wife would often become quite incensed, mentioning her husband's rank. This is where I learned that everyone in the military, right up to the Commander-in-Chief, has to answer to someone. So, when this situation arose, I would ask for the name of their serviceman husband's commander while moving toward the telephone as if I was planning to call. Suddenly, the patient would say that wouldn't be necessary (fearing a black mark on her husband's record that might preclude further promotion) and she would accede to my medical advice. Playing out that bluff was annoying, but all too often it was necessary. It was also a good learning experience for me because, although the colonels outranked me, it taught me not to be bullied into giving inappropriate care.

While most of the time I was treating common illnesses, I did see instances of unusual conditions. One experience occurred on a trip I took with a few of my medical colleagues via a Marine helicopter to a small outlying island that was the site of a leper colony. It was partially a goodwill mission to deliver donated clothing our wives gathered and also to study a fascinating medical problem. I had studied leprosy (Hansen's disease), in medical school, but thought I would never actually see a case. Leprosy is caused by a spirochete bacillus or bacteria and it causes two different forms of the disease—a nodular appearing skin disease, or a flat diffuse erythematous rash. The nodular form is particularly destructive and, on this trip, I saw people without fingers or with only a half a foot bilaterally. As a physician I was intrigued at seeing the disease in person, but I was also saddened to see the terrible physical and emotional effects it had on this group of people. Even, as in biblical times, these people were treated as outcasts because of their deformities, as well as the possibility of infectious transmission. They were grateful for our mission, but as we boarded our helicopter to depart, I imagine they wished they could leave as well.

As for serious cases I treated on the base, there were a few I remember very well. In the first, a young officer's wife came to the dispensary and was assigned to see me because she had an elevated temperature and felt ill. Examination revealed that she had a severely swollen and infected distal phalanx of the middle finger of her right-hand, which is called a felon. I was sure that this was the etiology of her fever and I knew that she would require antibiotics, but surgical drainage of the felon was also required. I checked the surgical textbook in the library to find out the appropriate method of drainage. It indicated that the tip of the finger should be incised in a fish-mouth manner to relieve the pressure caused by the swelling and to allow drainage of the purulent infected material. Unfortunately, the surgical text that I had consulted was out of date (drainage should have been done with a stab wound from side-to-side and placement of an iodoform gauze drain through the opening). I proceeded, based on the book's instructions, and the patient did improve. Her fever disappeared, the swelling went down, and there was a general improvement in her well-being. I saw her on a daily basis and after she was adequately recovered I was faced with what to do about the fish mouth incision that I had created. I elected to suture the distal aspect of the tip of the finger, leaving the sides open with a drain in-place and gradually allowing it to heal. This was a lengthy process but eventually the drain was removed and further suture closure carried out. She was left with a scar as well as some residual swelling. Toward the end of our daily visits I asked this woman if she had any hobbies or outside interests. She told me that prior to marrying her serviceman husband she was a concert pianist. It was then I realized that I should have asked her for this information as part of her earliest exam. Perhaps I would have wisely transferred her to a surgeon a few miles away instead of treating her myself.

Another case, somewhat similar to the previous, where I was again taught a lesson in humility took place one evening while I was the M.O.D. A sergeant was brought in to the dispensary emergency room after amputating the distal end of his finger when it was slammed and trapped in the large sliding metal door of an airplane hangar. The personnel working with him retrieved the tip of the finger and brought it in, appropriately, in a bucket of ice. There was a good deal in the medical literature about reattachment of fingers and limbs if the procedure could be accomplished quickly after the amputation and if the amputated part was appropriately preserved in a cooling solution or ice. I inspected the amputated finger and felt that reattachment was possible. I sutured the tip of the finger back on to the hand but realized

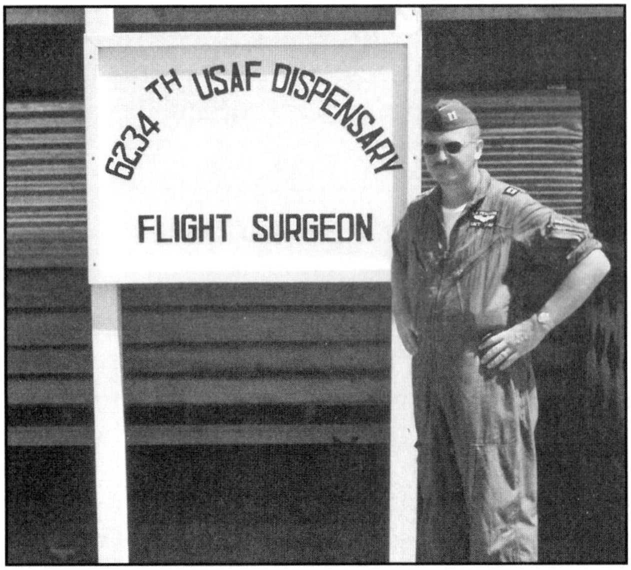

that a good deal of crush injury had occurred with splintering of the bone. I should have stopped right at that point and transferred the patient to the surgery service at the Army hospital at Kue for a definitive clean amputation. But I elected to suture the tip back on, minus the fingernail, which had been avulsed. The patient was treated with a tetanus booster shot, pain medication, and antibiotics. Evidence of viability over the next several days with growth of new blood vessels especially into the nail bed was present and I was somewhat encouraged by the result. However, this viability did not extend onto the pad of the finger and it became evident after several days that this area was not viable and becoming gangrenous. The patient therefore was sent to the surgical service for definitive amputation.

The third case that I recall vividly is the night I was on-call as the M.O.D. (on a Saturday) when our corpsmen were notified of a situation in the village of Koza that bordered Kadena Air Force Base. They quickly dispatched an Air Force ambulance to the area. I was soon notified that the patient was in the ambulance and corpsmen were administering resuscitative measures to a pulseless non-breather. When the ambulance arrived at our emergency area I was told the patient was a young Marine who was involved in an altercation in the village with other Marines and one of them had stabbed him. This conflict had probably been initiated by an argument over a “B-girl” working in one of the multiple sleazy nightclubs that seem to be attracted to military bases like bears to honey. Upon arrival a quick assessment was made of the patient and there were no signs of life. Because of his young age I felt that every effort possible should be made to try to revive him. Our resuscitative efforts went on for more than half an hour without result. There had been reports in the medical literature that opening the chest and massaging the heart directly might restore function. I elected to proceed with this approach as a last resort. I opened the chest with a scalpel incising between ribs on the left lateral thorax. As the thoracic cavity was entered a very large amount of blood flushed out onto the floor, already formed in a gelatinous clot, indicating that it was not fresh active bleeding. At this point, any further efforts at resuscitation were felt to be totally futile and the patient was pronounced dead. Because he was military and in view of the circumstances of receiving his fatal wound, I arranged for the patient to be transferred to the Kue Army Hospital for an autopsy. The Marine base and its commander were made aware of the situation and were in full agreement with my recommendations. It was determined at autopsy that the patient was stabbed with a stiletto type knife which left only a very small entry wound directly over his heart and that the knife had penetrated both the right and left atrium of the heart leading to death by exsanguination (blood loss). I did not know what measures were taken against his attackers until some time later when I received a phone call from the military police at the Marine base requesting that I be available to testify at the court-martial of the perpetrators of the fatal stabbing. I had no choice but to agree as I was under military orders to be present at the trial. On the appointed day a military Jeep with two military policemen came to the dispensary to transport me to the proceedings. In due time I was sworn in and placed in the witness chair in front of the court-martial panel. I related my involvement on that fateful night and then responded to questions from the panel and from the defense counsel. I was asked whether it was possible that in opening the chest with my scalpel I had created the wound in the heart and had been responsible for the patient's demise. I was completely convinced that this was a total impossibility and so testified, but it did give me pause to reflect on my role in this scenario, and how close I was to becoming a defendant rather than a witness. The court accepted my explanation and without further questioning dismissed me. I was escorted back to my duty station by the same military police in their Jeep. I never did find out the disposition of the court-martial nor the fate of the defendants. It is probably best that I did not know. I did have great empathy for them and an understanding of what an impulsive act can bring about in the flash of a moment. I remember looking into the eyes of the two young Marines on trial and I observed them as typical young adults, clean cut, muscular and hardened by their training, and in all other respects other than the unfortunate act they were accused of, they were the epitome of what one would visualize as the ideal fighting man and Marine. That visual impression remains with me to this day.

On duty as the M.O.D., late one evening, I was presented with a sick child brought in by his young parents. The child was about one-year-old and their first child and therefore they had a heightened parental concern. The child was ill with symptoms of an upper respiratory infection and was febrile. I made a very careful examination and took the appropriate cultures and blood counts and prescribed decongestants and anti-fever medications. I don't know why, but maybe I was developing that sixth-sense of observation and concern that leads physicians to "smell trouble". I felt the child was more irritable when handled or held than the usual sick child with a respiratory illness. The child definitely did not have a stiff neck (nuchal rigidity) but became more fussy and irritable with any movement, neck or otherwise. I told the parents I was concerned that the child could be showing early signs of meningitis but the findings were not conclusive at this time. We as physicians and as parents have all seen young kids who seem to be extremely ill and become febrile very quickly but with symptomatic treatment turn right around and act like nothing is wrong a few hours later. I instructed the parents to take the child home and administer the medications prescribed but if the child was no better in two hours to let me know. They called back, probably no more than one hour later, stating the child was no better and in fact looked worse. I instructed them to take the child immediately to the Kue Army Hospital and not to come back to see me. I told them I would call ahead so that the physicians there were prepared to take care of the child immediately. The parents did as I said and very prompt attention by the physicians at Kue including a spinal tap quickly confirmed the child did, in fact, have meningitis. In spite of intravenous antibiotics, the child quickly deteriorated and died before morning. Although there was probably nothing that I could have done that would have saved the child's life, nevertheless, I felt a deep despair and one of those "would've, could've, should've" moments of self-flagellation.

Once again, on duty as the M.O.D. in the early evening, a car came speeding into the parking lot behind the dispensary near the emergency entrance, slammed on the brakes and skidded to a stop. A very frightened and anxious mother jumped out of the car and grabbed her daughter, probably age four, out of the passenger seat and rushed in the door with her, in a panic. The young girl had inhaled a small ceramic bathroom tile from a deteriorated shower wall in an off-base house where they lived. The tile actually had entered the larynx just above the vocal cords and with each breath the child took it was acting like a flap valve obstructing the airway. This of course made a rather "crowing" sound with each respiration that frightened the mother and led to her correct assessment of the problem. Fortunately, enough air was able to get into the trachea and lungs to avoid suffocation. With help from my corpsmen and with gentle restraint I was able to visualize the tile with a laryngoscope and extract it with a long armed forceps or hemostat. Fortunately, the piece of tile was standing on end as the forceps approached it and it was easy to grasp and extract. The frightened child quickly returned to her normal self and the mother broke down in tears of relief. I reassured her the problem was over and she could take her child home, but advised that they insist that their landlord repair the shower area of their home. She left the parking lot calmer than when she had entered. It was a moment of gratification for me and I was thankful I was successful in removing this foreign body.

My military service came to an end in mid-April 1966. It was time to move on. I found it to be a very difficult decision to leave the Air Force. For the past three years, stationed on a pacific island, 60 miles long and 2-18 miles wide, my wife and I had enjoyed the camaraderie and social life with our fellow physicians, dentists, lawyers, aircrew members, and their families, as well as developing a strong relationship with an Okinawan family. I can truly say that these were some of the best years of my life.

At this point in my career I decided it was most appropriate for me to enter a residency program in Internal Medicine because I felt I had forgotten a lot of what I had learned in the past about taking care of very sick patients. Therefore, I wrote to two of my classmates who were residents in training at Milwaukee County General Hospital and asked if they could recommend me to the staff as a potential resident in that specialty. They were more than happy to do so and after appropriate applications were completed I was offered a position as a first-year resident in Internal Medicine.

I returned to the United States and was discharged from the United States Air Force at Travis Air Force Base in California. The biggest initial adjustment was the 14-hour time differential. We soon returned to Wisconsin and became reacquainted with family and friends who also met our two-year-old daughter, Linda, for the first time. Prior to leaving Okinawa I ordered a new car through communication with my dad. When we arrived in Wisconsin, a powder blue 1966 Mustang was waiting for us at Wendt Ford in Waupaca, WI.

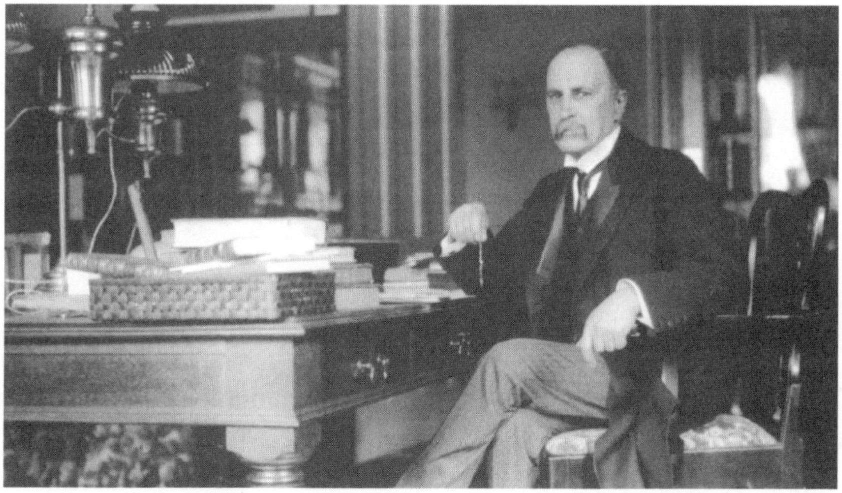

"The practice of medicine is an art, not a trade, a calling, not a business; a calling in which your heart will be exercised equally with your head."

—Sir William Osler

Chapter Nine

INTERNAL MEDICINE RESIDENCY

(1966-1969)

I began my internal medicine residency program at Milwaukee County General Hospital in June 1966. My first assignment was to the pulmonary tuberculosis service which, strangely, still had an adequate number of patients to merit its own ward. The new anti-TB drugs discovered in the 1950s were effectively treating this age-old scourge and the TB sanitariums that had checker-boarded the entire country through the 1940s were closing or were very sparsely populated. In view of my absence from a hospital setting for the past three years, I was glad to have a gentle month-long reintroduction into the world of academic and bedside medicine on a service that was not involved in intense acute care. TB is rather straightforward in terms of its transmission. The Mycobacterium bacilli (TB bacterial organisms) are disseminated from person-to-person via cough-initiated airborne particles and the disease then presents as an active primary infection of the lungs, although it can affect almost any organ of the body, including the skeleton. It may cause acute or subacute respiratory disease with symptoms of cough, fever, malaise, weight-loss, and hemoptysis (coughing up blood)—or, after the primary infection, may lie dormant and reactivate many years later. Nevertheless, TB is a deadly disease. When I saw patients on the ward with debilitating lung disease, or whose adrenal glands had been destroyed leaving them with life-threatening Addison's disease, or when I evaluated those who had developed scrofula (involvement of the lymph nodes of the neck by TB), or Pott's Disease—a vertebra destroying TB disease of the spine—I realized how much I had forgotten about TB and infectious diseases in general.

At one point, a febrile, dehydrated TB patient suddenly went into diabetic ketoacidosis with a massive rise in serum blood sugar which caused osmotic diuresis (urine flow stimulated by the supersaturated serum glucose bombarding the kidneys) leading to further dehydration and electrolyte imbalance. I remembered learning about this condition in med school but I had forgotten how to treat it, and to my surprise, my pulmonary professor in charge of the TB ward did not remember either! Ironically, the senior medical students who were under my supervision understood my dilemma and my frustration. They had been well educated about this disease in the classroom and had previous experience in treating this condition. One said, "Don't worry, Doc. We'll talk you through it." And they did. I was completely embarrassed and humbled, but believe me, that night I got out a book on diagnosis and treatment and studied. From that time forward, that book was near at hand and when I faced a situation I did not understand completely, I retreated to study and refresh my memory. Not surprisingly, I also came to the very wise conclusion that only egomaniacs or idiots would shut out their interns and medical students and relegate them to being mere observers. Unfortunately, I had experienced enough of that during my internship, leaving me unprepared to handle the current problem. Henceforth, I always tried to involve my team in the decision making such that we served as sounding boards for each other to the benefit of the patient.

I soon began to feel at ease in the hospital setting, which was fortunate because my next rotation was the management of a general medical ward. The medical wards at the county hospital were designed to hold 20 patients with eight beds on each side of an open ward and four private rooms for the most seriously ill. Often, the census swelled to 25 or 30 patients, with overflow beds placed down the middle aisle of the open ward and on a sun porch at the end of the ward. It was a scene transposed, without change, right out of the hospitals of the European Middle Ages! On the open wards, curtains or temporary screens separated the beds—not even close to the most unsophisticated version of privacy.

I was on night-call every other day and weekend-call every other weekend. At night, the resident was responsible for two wards of male patients or two wards of female patients, and took all of the admissions. Without the able assistance of the two interns and two senior students on my team, my job would have been intolerable. I think I still hold the record for the most admissions in a 24-hour period: a total of 26 patients, some of which went to the intensive care unit. I was so exhausted by the time we admitted the last patient at 5 a.m., everything I did was purely robotic. Fortunately for me, the very last person to come in did not require much more than perfunctory care: it was a young healthy appearing lady who had overdosed on barbiturates and was comatose in her drug-induced deep sleep, but who was breathing normally and had stable vital signs. I immediately plugged in IVs in both arms and opened them up to run wide open, placed a catheter in her bladder to drain off the fluid as it flushed the drugs from her system, and then announced that I was going to bed. I crawled onto a nearby cot and told the nurses to awaken me if there were any problems. As expected, the woman's recovery proceeded without incident and I was able to get a couple of hours of sleep before I had to start another day of patient care and admissions.

I know that today there are many young resident doctors who still work long hours, but the exorbitant work demands of my era have been modified because of concerns for patient safety and to avoid errors made by sleep-deprived trainees. However, there is one other significant difference between working on the wards then and now: in the 1960s, many (or most) health care facilities were without air conditioning. I recall that during summer heat waves the nursing homes throughout Milwaukee would unleash a steady stream of ambulance runs to our hospital, delivering a population of severely dehydrated, elderly patients. Most of them were already comatose and exhibiting the "O" sign (in which the mouth is wide open in an "O" shape, and the person is mouth-breathing, hyperventilating, and struggling for air). One Sunday in early July I was on-call, and, I remember the temperature hovering around 100° F. with humidity that made me feel like I needed gills to survive. Patient after patient arrived with high respiratory rates, parched mucous membranes of the mouth, and high body temperatures. Their skin was doughy with poor turgor (a sign of dehydration in which the skin remains tented when pinched instead of snapping back to normal). As IVs were started, fever control initiated, Foley catheters placed in the bladder (often dry as a bone at the start), and antibiotics administered when necessary, I would then go on to administer similar care to the next patient, and the next. At least I didn't have to waste time eliciting a medical history from a comatose patient. Eventually they would wake up, start passing urine, stabilize their vital signs, and recover enough to return to the nursing home the next day. We tried to lessen the oppressive heat, but opening the windows and positioning fans around the ward did little to help. My short-sleeve, white dress shirt and white trousers were totally soaked and the sweat ran off my face in rivulets. I hadn't sweat that profusely since my summers working in the haymow back on the farm. I will never forget how incredibly relieved I was when, later in the day, a freak cold front went through. The temperature plummeted about 40 degrees and left me shivering in my wet clothes. Severe thunderstorms and tornado warnings followed, but, like the patients, the weather stabilized over the next several hours and things returned to normal.

The experience on the wards at the VA (Veterans Administration) hospital was quite different from that at MCGH. The wards had 20 beds, a number that was never exceeded. A new patient could not be admitted until one was discharged. The federal funding of the hospital was granted according to its ability to keep the beds full. Therefore, our turnover was usually no more than four or five patients per day. One of my friends, Terry Moritz, clearly did not realize this modus operandi because on the first day of his ward service he concluded that most of the patients were ready for discharge, so he let them go. This nearly empty ward created chaos and summoned a visit from the chief of medicine, who informed Terry that this was not how the VA worked. Another quirk of the VA was that it had its own hired physicians who were responsible for half of the wards, but they only worked during the day, and we, as residents covered their wards at night. On one occasion, one of these M.D.s was in the initial treatment of a severely-ill diabetic patient in ketoacidosis. When 5 p.m. rolled around, he left! Because the patient was still comatose, I spent the next several hours trying to stabilize him. I was angry and could not believe what I had just seen. It was not my mindset to walk out on a critically-ill patient, and I vowed that I would never do that.

Another instance that dumbfounded me came courtesy of a head nurse on my ward at the VA. She was young, blond, wore a white starched uniform and nurse's cap (something that is never seen today), and sported a huge diamond engagement ring on her finger. She was my own personal Nurse Cratchet (if you remember, *One Flew Over The Cuckoo's Nest*). An example of her air-head, dumb-blond (cliché—I have nothing against blonds), incompetence that I remember (I'm sure I have blocked out others) occurred when I was treating a patient with pneumonia who had a fever of 105° F. with probable acute sepsis (systemic infection through the blood stream). A cooling blanket was placed on the patient and I wrote the order to reduce the patient's body temperature to 101° F. With the blanket, antipyretics (fever lowering meds), IV fluids, and the beneficial effect of antibiotics the patient's temperature returned to a completely normal 98.6° F. The nurse saw this and responded by turning the blanket to "heat" in order to raise the patient's temperature to 101° F. I could barely control my rage, and I wondered, sympathetically, in subsequent weeks about the unsuspecting boyfriend who had given her the big ring. I felt sorry for him.

In sharp contrast to the incompetent nurse were the many positive experiences during the residency. Numerous visiting professors from Harvard, New York Mount Sinai, Georgetown, George Washington University, and elsewhere came to MCGH to give lectures, do Grand Rounds discussions in the auditorium, or to meet with the house-staff regarding interesting cases on the wards. The most interesting and, in my mind, the most awesome of all of these guests was Dr. Linus Pauling, winner of the Nobel Prize in chemistry and also the Nobel Peace Prize. He discovered Vitamin C (and personally took a megadose of 16 grams daily for 30 years prior to his death at age 96). To listen to him speak and discuss his research and to talk to him personally was a mind-boggling experience. It was also the first time I felt star-struck by someone in the medical research profession, which was odd and exhilarating at the same time. To sit at the feet of scholars, geniuses, and Nobel Laureates is one of the most rewarding educational experiences anyone can imagine and to have it all wrapped up in one individual was truly exceptional.

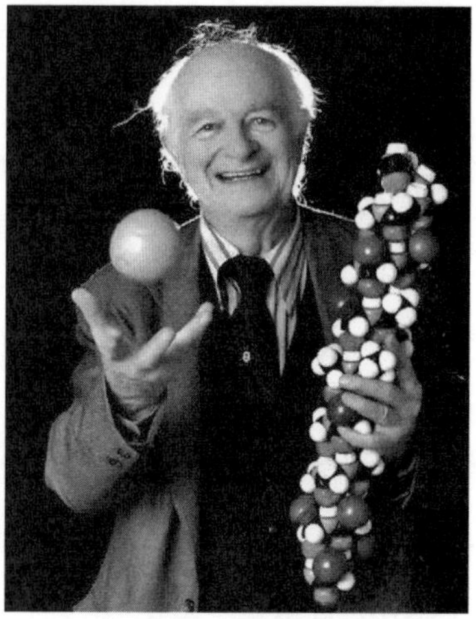

Dr. Linus Pauling with an orange and a chemical model of Vitamin C

The once-in-a-lifetime chance to hear Dr. Pauling and be exposed to other scholarly professors was certainly a highlight of my training, but, on a daily basis, the learning experience came from the varied array of medical conditions I treated at MCGH. Up to this point in my career I had been in contact with rather homogeneous populations of patients in private or community hospitals, or in outpatient clinics. At MCGH, however, we had a wide spectrum of patients, both in economic status and ethnicity. For example, we served a very large black population and, therefore, I suddenly needed to become familiar with treating Sickle Cell Anemia, which is a genetic condition that is fairly common in African-Americans. Sickle Cell disease deforms red blood cells and this may result in intravascular clot formation, as well as a Sickle Cell Crisis, which may be a life-threatening hemolytic (red blood cell destroying) anemia. I also found it difficult to understand why the blacks and the poor also often exhibited extraordinary prevalence of obesity, (and paradoxically), malnutrition, vitamin and iron deficiency, and insulin-dependent diabetes, which made their associated renal, liver, and heart disease very difficult to treat. Many blacks, men and women, who had emigrated to Milwaukee from the South, had a practice of chewing a certain type of southern clay as if it were tobacco—a condition medically known as, a Pica Syndrome. This, by some means, can cause severe anemia. I came to realize that I had to adjust to understanding their culture, lifestyle, unique medical conditions, and socio-economic status rather than trying to make them conform to my preconceived notions of pervading social and medical attitudes.

In addition to the patients, the hospital staff came from all walks of life, and while we all worked very well together, occasionally situations arose where I would become very conscious of the fact that this was really my first time working and socializing with people who had different social and economic backgrounds. One Friday afternoon after work, the resident and intern house-staff, not on night-call, made our usual pit stop at a quaint little bar next to the railroad tracks, not far from the county hospital. Unlike other Fridays, however, this time several of our black nurse's aides (presumably invited by members of the house-staff) came over for happy hour as well. At this time, bars were relatively segregated based on their neighborhood. Everyone had a great time and after several rounds of drinks and the usual exchange of macabre medical humor, the aides invited us to go with them to their neighborhood hangout. Not wanting the good times to end, a few of us agreed, and we were off. Very quickly after arriving, however, I became uneasy as I saw other patrons and the bartender looking apprehensively at us, the only white people in the place. I wondered if the women who came to our bar felt the same discomfort when they were the only black people there. In any event, I was getting the idea that our presence might be disruptive. I told one aide, the ironically named, Miss White, that I thought maybe it would be best if we left. She said, "Don't worry. Nobody is going to mess with you." I admitted, that yes, I thought someone might mess with me. She said, "No chance," and she opened her purse to show me a silver-plated revolver. That's when I was certain it was time to leave and I was out the door and on my way home in a flash. The house-staff and the aides continued to have a friendly rapport at work, but never again did either group venture past their own comfort zones. I could say that our insecurities and reactions were just related to the times, (an era of civil rights marches, MLK, LA-Watts burning, riots, curfews, etc.), but our attitudes may not be much different today.

❤

Any physician who has served in a residency program at a city or county hospital in a large metropolitan area can relate unending stories of bizarre, interesting, tragic, comical, and rewarding experiences they encountered on duty in the emergency room. I would like to present several interesting cases that stand out in my mind from my ER experience at MCGH.

A frequent female visitor to the emergency room, was borderline psychotic and certainly hysterical. On one occasion, she faked a fainting episode and lay on the floor in the flow of traffic to gain attention. A resident saw her, recognized her, and quickly resolved the situation by stating, "lunch is served." She promptly became conscious, rose to her feet, and asked directions to the lunchroom. This same patient arrived in the emergency room one evening and told the doctor that she had a mouth full of razor blades and would swallow them if he did not admit her to the hospital. The surgery resident, Dr. Aprahamian, tired and overworked, said to her, "Dammit, either swallow them or spit them out; I don't have time to put up with your BS." She left without further ado—after spitting out two razor blades.

A very strong, young, black man had multiple admissions to the emergency room due to alcoholic delirium tremens (DTs). He required a full set of leather arm and body restraints as well as marked sedation to prevent him from injuring himself or others as he fought against the demons that he saw attacking him from the walls and ceilings. I actually saw him, in full leather restraints with his wrists tethered to the side of the gurney, suddenly grasp the railings of the cart with his hands and bend them right in upon himself. I stood there in amazement and quickly decided that I better be very careful when I examined him. I had visions of him strangling me with one hand or grabbing my stethoscope and pulling the ears right off my head. He was kept in an observation room under sedation until he became rational and then he was discharged and escorted home by the county sheriff's deputies. He returned to the ER many times escorted by those same deputies when his violent and irrational behavior was again manifest after an alcoholic binge and withdrawal period.

A man was brought to the ER by the police with a GSW (gunshot wound). This was a shotgun wound that had resulted in multiple pellets entering his thighs. He tried to convince us it was an accident, but the police officers accompanying him quickly informed us not to believe it. They stated that he had tried to enter the house of his estranged wife or girlfriend at 5 a.m. and she blasted him with a shotgun burst right through the door panels. I don't think she was aiming for his legs. Fortunately, the door panel took the brunt of the blast and the pellets in his legs were quite superficial and easily removed.

In the middle of the winter, a homeless man was brought to the emergency room from an abandoned unheated building. When his slush-soaked shoes (without socks) were removed from his feet, the soles of his feet came off with the shoes. He was admitted to the hospital and because of his filthy status, the nurse's aides put him directly in the shower, clothes and all. After a good soaking they removed his clothes, bagged them to be burned, scrubbed him with soap and brushes, and treated his skin and hair with delousing powder. He was discharged to a temporary shelter facility where he was given donated shoes and clothes. As was usual with many homeless, he probably wandered off and went right back to his unheated abandoned warehouse. The homeless, sleeping under bridges or on sewer grates for the heat, were frequent winter visitors to the county hospital after humanitarily being picked up for vagrancy by the city and county police.

Two black men were admitted to the hospital via the emergency room after entering with gunshot wounds (GSWs) from handguns. The story was that four men became embroiled in an argument at a bar on the near north side of Milwaukee. I was flabbergasted when I took their history and found out that they collectively made a decision, rationally or irrationally, to go home, get their handguns and shoot it out on the street. When they returned, each took position on the four corners of an intersection and opened fire. Two of them were wounded by gunfire, but I was afraid to ask what happened to the other two. The two wounded men were placed in the hospital and handcuffed to their beds under armed guard. Because the county could only spare one deputy to watch both, they were placed in the same room, foot-to-foot, in their separate beds. Twenty-four hours later, amazingly, they were still sitting up in bed threatening each other with great bodily harm. (How irrational is that?) They went to jail directly from the hospital, hopefully defusing the situation at least for the time being.

One day, I was consulting on a patient on the urology service when I heard a din of uproarious laughter coming from the office of the chief urology resident. I decided to check it out and found several residents and nurses viewing an X-ray of a young teenage boy who had been admitted from the emergency room during the night with inability to urinate. An X-ray revealed his bladder was packed full of .22 caliber shells he had systematically passed, one after the other, through his penis into his bladder. Needless to say, following opening of his bladder surgically and removing the bullets, the patient was transferred to the psychiatric service.

♥

Because of their rather complex and challenging medical conditions, the following cases, although admitted via the ER, were cared for by my team and me on the medical ward.

A female patient in a semi-comatose state was driven to the hospital by her husband. Her electrolyte blood tests on admission were very abnormal with sodium, potassium, and chlorides all extremely low. It is said as an axiom that if the sodium in the blood is less than 105 (normal: 140-145), survival is unlikely. Hers was 102. There are several possible causes for this. A condition called Diabetes Insipidus, a pituitary gland hormone problem can cause this situation, as can Primary Hyperaldosteronism, an adrenal gland abnormality. After interviewing her husband, I learned that they had been in a prolonged and heated argument when she became less and less coherent. He also noted that on the way to the hospital she had vomited a large amount of clear watery liquid. On further careful questioning, I determined that during the argument she frequently went to the sink and drank glasses of water. Therefore, the diagnosis became clear that the patient was a "Psychogenic Water Drinker" and under conditions of stress utilized this way of handling the situation, intoxicating herself with water in the process. The treatment I provided gradually returned her electrolytes to normal, she became fully conscious, and arrangements were made for a psychiatric evaluation.

A male on our ward was very ill, but his symptoms and physical signs by examination were unusually strange and kept changing. He continued to exhibit a progressive deterioration. At first I thought it might be psychiatric hysteria, but as he continued to fail I considered rare medical diseases. Because he began to have unusual neurological findings, the neurology service was consulted. They were also quite puzzled for several days but finally pinned the diagnosis down with a blood-screening exam for heavy metals that revealed a high concentration of arsenic. His seemingly loving wife had insisted on assisting in feeding him at least twice per day. With clandestine observation, she was observed to be spiking his coffee with a powdery substance. The patient made only a partial recovery and was sent to a nursing home while the wife was escorted to jail.

I have an unforgettable memory of a patient who died on my ward during the night. The patient was admitted to the hospital on so many occasions that she was well known to all the residents. Her medical record consisted of multiple volumes that probably weighed more than ten pounds. On this admission she was almost comatose and her vital signs were failing rapidly. It was the patient's wish to have no further heroic measures carried out, but the intern and I did try to stabilize her blood pressure, pulse rate, and respiration with the use of intravenous medications. In spite of this it appeared that death was imminent and she lapsed deeper into coma. Attempts were made to contact her family and make them aware of her pre-terminal status. Finally, a son returned our telephone call which was answered by my intern. At the same time he was explaining the situation to the son on the telephone, I was listening to the patient's heart with my stethoscope and clearly heard each heartbeat as the pulse rate slowed and eventually stopped and no heartbeat was detectable. Respiration ceased. After a minute or two of observation I stepped out of the room and told my intern that the patient had expired, which he relayed to her son, who said "thank you", and hung up. I returned to the patient's room to make the official pronouncement of the patient's death by checking for pulse, respiration, response to painful stimuli, and checking the pupils, finding them fixed and dilated. No sign of life appeared to be present. I then placed my stethoscope back over the patient's heart and, much to my amazement, I heard a single heartbeat which was followed multiple seconds later with another heartbeat, and then the heart rate gradually increased over the next few minutes to normal and the patient began very shallow respirations. I was flabbergasted and quickly had a very horrible feeling in my stomach. With the intravenous medications continuing, her heartbeat and respirations became stronger and she regained a blood pressure. After moments of indecision, I knew what I had to do, and I went to the telephone and called her son to explain to him that there had been a mistake and that his mother had not expired. Again, he very blandly said, "thank you," with no evidence of recrimination in his voice. I then asked him if he was going to come to the hospital to see his mother. He said no, he had no interest in getting out of bed to come to see her. He stated that she had never done anything for him. I hung up the phone with a great sadness in my heart. No one should have to die alone no matter what grievance a family member might have toward the afflicted. I sat by this lady's bedside, comforting myself as much as her, for the next two hours, fully realizing and aware that her situation was irrecoverable and pre-mortem. Later, the patient deteriorated again and expired quietly with me at the bedside as her only mourner. After a much longer waiting period, I pronounced her dead for the second time. As the sun rose, I again called her son to report to him the time of death and inform him the hospital would contact him for further disposition of her remains. He again said, "thank you", without emotion and hung up. I can truthfully say, that in all my years of practicing medicine since that time, I have never encountered a similar reaction by the next of kin. Often, in contrast, an estranged relationship that ends in death results in a significant guilt trip and a desire by the family member to make amends by being overly attentive. I did learn from this experience that I should not be hasty in pronouncing someone dead, no matter what the circumstances. After all, they are not going anywhere any time soon.

A retired schoolteacher, quite elderly, but seemingly in quite good physical condition for her age and mentally clear and alert, was admitted at the request of her family because they were no longer able to care for her. The reason given for placing her in a care facility was that she had periods of confusion. Although the patient appeared to have quite a good handle on reality during daytime hours, at night she became totally psychotic, a condition well known to the medical profession, which in colloquial terms is called "sundowning". Over the years, as a teacher she apparently traveled to ply her profession in various schools, making these trips by train, and she was now reliving those experiences during the nights on my ward. This, needless to say, was very disruptive for the other patients. She would talk all night long in a very loud voice, calling for the conductor to provide her with some amenity. I can still hear her, "Conductor, Conductor, Conductor—" (and on and on). I can almost imagine the conductors were as distressed and annoyed then as we were now. About the only antipsychotic medication available to us was Thorazine®, and I prescribed this for her two or three times per night. This allowed her to rest, so that the rest of the ward could also get some rest. After several days and no nursing home bed in sight, it was noted on our morning rounds that she was becoming jaundiced. Because she also complained of stomach upset and abdominal pain, I became quite concerned that she had a gallbladder problem, either acute gallbladder inflammation, or a gallstone obstructing the common duct leading to the intestine. A surgical consultation was obtained from a senior surgical resident who agreed with this diagnosis and took her to surgery where he found a totally normal gallbladder and no evidence of stones. In those days there were no ultrasounds, CT scans, or MRIs to assist with confirmation of our clinical impression. We only had our physical examination, clinical experience, and laboratory tests to rely on. Surgical and medical staff physicians reviewed the case and decided her jaundice was most likely related to toxic effects from her Thorazine® therapy. In retrospect, this now seemed quite obvious, and the surgery resident and I were humbled by the experience. The patient unexplainably died several days later, presumably related to her age, an acute cardiac event, the stress of the surgery, and her ongoing hyperactive confusional state, which was no longer able to be treated by sedative drugs. If one could ever say "this was her time," I guess one could not refute it.

On a Saturday night I admitted two relatively young, black, female patients from the emergency room to my ward for treatment of their heroin drug addiction and associated problems. I started them on a methadone protocol to gradually wean them from their narcotic addiction. I really did not mind having them on my ward as they were considerably younger than any of my other patients, were pleasant and cooperative, jovial, and did not have any serious complication of their habit. The following morning, on Sunday, I arrived on the ward to make rounds and was soon made aware by the nurses that something odd was going on with these new patients. The drapes had been pulled around their beds obscuring visualization of them from the nurse's station or other areas on the ward. They also had male visitors early in the morning, also unusual, and there was a good deal of laughing, talking, and generalized jocularity coming from their adjoining beds and the area behind the drapes. I soon surmised that the male visitors had brought in drugs and the girls were shooting these drugs into their system right on my ward. I was dumbfounded, and felt that I had been duped. I pulled the drapes back and insisted that they remain open, and in no uncertain terms, chased the visitors off the ward and out of the hospital, threatening them with law enforcement intervention if they returned. The patients, now high on their drugs again, were oblivious to any concerns going on around them. I was concerned about my legal responsibility. Could I be accused of harboring addicts and abetting their illegal acts? I called the detective bureau of the Milwaukee County justice system and talked with a detective. After explaining the situation as noted above, he advised me that I had no personal concerns or legal responsibilities. Being much more familiar with this shady world than I, he explained to me that it was likely that my girl patients were prostitutes and their male attendants that I scurried from the hospital were their pimps who kept them supplied with drugs and therefore enslaved. I was astounded! He went on to say, when a prostitute's drug habit becomes too expensive such that they can't support it with their income from the world's oldest profession, they need treatment, not for a cure, but to reduce their dependence on the costly illegal drugs. The detective advised me that it was likely that they would sign themselves out of the hospital AMA, (against medical advice) when their drug dependency needs had been weaned to a point they could afford. He was totally correct. The experience, which in today's culture might be less mind-boggling, had, at that time, made me a bit more streetwise.

In the 1960s, the only diuretics that we had available for treating intra- or extravascular (inside or outside the blood vessels) fluid overload, were oral thiazides or intramuscular injections of mercurial diuretics, which were only mildly effective. The medical condition of "dropsy" or severe swelling (edema) of the lower extremities was very prevalent and was usually related to the heart's inability to pump blood well (congestive heart failure) or the kidneys inability to clear the excess water volume by urination (renal insufficiency). The legs would sometimes become so edematous that the skin couldn't hold the fluid, causing it to break down and weep. In older days, doctors made incisions in the skin of the legs to allow more fluid drainage. I had a patient on my ward, totally bedridden with such severe edema that it involved her entire body, a condition called anasarca. The pitiful helplessness—and yes, probable hopelessness—which I experienced in my heart was profound as I tried my best to treat her condition with whatever means were available to me. But one day, I called a staff doctor from the renal service to consult on this very unfortunate lady. He reviewed what we were doing for her and approved of our fluid and salt restriction, digitalis to strengthen the heart's contraction, and the gentle diuretics. He then said that he had just received a supply of a brand-new diuretic drug from a pharmaceutical company for trial in a clinical setting. The consultant felt that, based on the information he had, it just might help my patient. The renal staff doctor did not know much about the drug and we knew nothing about it. He was told by the company that they thought the dosage should be 100 mg twice a day and that giving the entire dose of 200 mg all at once got better results than splitting the dosage. The drug was called ethycrinic acid. I could hardly wait to get my hands on this possible miracle drug. The staff doctor went to his laboratory and came back with a vial of the drug, and in our desperation, I administered 200 mg intramuscularly. Within minutes the patient experienced a need to void, so, because of her large size, we helped her onto a bedside commode. She began to void and literally did not stop passing urine for hours. It was one of the most amazing things I experienced in my career. I had administered a very large dose of ethycrinic acid which she tolerated due to her large size, but, I learned that I had to be cautious in my dosing to avoid electrolyte abnormalities from occurring. This was the first of the so-called "loop-diuretics" that work directly on the tubules emanating from the glomeruli (filtration apparatus) of the kidney. Soon this drug became available in oral form and a second potent loop-diuretic, furosemide, was also available. I was thrilled to witness a miracle occur that would change the therapy of heart failure forever. It was a "Eureka!" moment in history.

♥

The following is background information for the next case presentation:

Dr. Waisbren of the infectious disease service was in private practice in Milwaukee but also was the titular head of the department of infectious diseases at MCGH, and was also on the staff of multiple hospitals throughout the city. He was somewhat of a radical, believing in megadoses of antibiotics often given in combination to cover every possibility. His usual cocktail of antibiotics for intravenous use consisted of 16 grams of penicillin, 16 grams of cephalosporin, and an equally hefty dose of kanamycin or gentamycin given daily. While I was on his service I did quite a bit of dog surgery, removing the kidneys from dogs that had been infected with E. coli or given progressive immunizing dosages of E. coli toxin. These kidneys were then evaluated in Dr. Waisbren's laboratory in an attempt to create an E. coli antitoxin. At that time I was certainly not aware of how deadly the E. coli toxin could be, but fortunately, I did not become exposed or ill. Because I was a farm boy, I reasoned that somehow dairy farmers who were constantly exposed to manure, and therefore E. coli, must build up a natural immunity to the toxin. Dr. Waisbren became very enthused with my theory and only somewhat jokingly indicated that he was sure that we could win the Nobel Prize if we could develop experimental evidence to support it. Of course, nothing ever came of this.

While I was on the Infectious Disease service a female patient was transferred from a community hospital in the eastern part of Wisconsin near Lake Michigan. A sliver from an old wooden post became embedded under a fingernail as she rebuilt a fence with her husband. The finger became infected and swollen and there were red streaks going up through the hand and forearm. In the course of her illness she developed significant trismus (spasm) of her facial and jaw muscles and spasms of generalized muscle contraction throughout her body. She was suffering from Tetanus or "Lockjaw", a systemic infection caused by a bacillus organism. She was treated with surgical debridement (open drainage and removal of non-viable tissue) of her infected finger, tetanus antitoxin, and large dose antibiotic cocktails of Dr. Waisbren's concoction. The muscle spasms that came in waves were partially controlled by muscle relaxant medications, narcotics, and intravenous Valium. Her case was discussed in great detail by multiple staff physicians at numerous conferences, but I was the one who was involved with the daily primary care of the patient as the resident on the infectious disease service. After several very taxing days of treatment, trying to buy time, hoping her intrinsic antibodies would come to the rescue, her situation deteriorated rapidly and she died. I am happy that I have never seen another case of this in my career.

❤

The next two cases that I am going to discuss will be presented in the format of a Clinical-Pathological-Conference (CPC). They are so unique and unusual that I think it is important to present them here, in abridged fashion, as they were presented to the staff and my fellow residents, interns, and students in the large Joseph King Auditorium of the hospital. I was intimately involved with these cases as the attending resident physician. I feel a bit of sadness today that the CPC is no longer used as a teaching tool. Today, so much information can be obtained technologically by Echo, MRI, CT scans, and other sophisticated means that the deductive reasoning, searching for clues in the presentation of a difficult case, is no longer necessary. In addition, autopsies are rarely used today for determination of the cause of death.

CPC Case Number One: The patient was a 48-year-old, obese, divorced black female who had been seen in the ER for bilateral epistaxis (nosebleeds). There was no past history of bleeding disorders and no previous history of hemorrhage. She was found to be hypertensive with a blood pressure of 240/120 and her pulse was irregular. Eight years prior to admission she was told she had hypertension and took medication for three months and then discontinued it. Her weight had been stable at 270 pounds for the past 20 years. Her mother had died at age 42 of a cerebral hemorrhage. Social history was interesting in that she had been Clark Gable's cook for several years prior to moving to the Milwaukee area. Physical examination revealed an alert, oriented, obese lady in no distress. Hypertensive changes of the blood vessels on the retina of the eyes were present. Carotid pulses were equal and normal without bruits. Lungs were clear. A grade I/VI systolic heart murmur was heard. Pedal pulses were strong and there was no edema. Deep tendon reflexes were equal bilaterally. Her hospital course consisted of therapy of her hypertension and treatment of a urinary tract infection. Blood pressure stabilized at about 140/90. Further X-rays and examination revealed a large staghorn calculus (stone) of the right kidney and poor visualization of the left kidney as well as a large pelvic mass felt to be a fibroid uterus. Several days following admission she had an episode of near syncope (fainting) and felt short of breath with tightness in her throat and was noted to be hyperventilating. Several days later she again appeared weak and short of breath and seemed to be confused. A sickle-cell preparation of her blood was positive. Sixteen days after admission she continued to have malaise, weakness, shortness of breath, intermittent abdominal pain, vomiting, belching, and hyperventilation to 48 respirations per minute. She complained of numbness and throbbing of the entire left leg but several examiners were unsure if there was evidence of thrombophlebitis (vein clots and inflammation). Intravenous heparin anticoagulation was started empirically. 24 hours later she was found in bed gasping, unresponsive, eyes rolled to the right, and then to the left, and then fixed centrally, followed closely by cardiac and respiratory arrest that did not respond to resuscitation efforts and she was pronounced dead.

Pathologic diagnosis of Case Number One: The patient showed evidence of recurrent pulmonary emboli (clots in the lungs) that probably had occurred throughout her hospitalization. The etiology of the emboli to her lungs was an active thrombophlebitis of the lower extremities with extensive clot formation that had probably been contributed to by her sickle cell disease as well as her extended period of bed rest during the evaluation and therapy of her severe hypertension. Her cerebral vascular accident (stroke) that led to her death was caused by paradoxical emboli that had passed from her right-sided venous circulation to the left-sided arterial circulation and thence to her brain via a large patent atrial septal defect of the heart.

CPC Case Number Two: A 27-year-old white female had delivered a term infant at an outlying hospital eight weeks prior to admission to Milwaukee County General Hospital. Prolonged postpartum bleeding, poorly responsive to ergotamine (capillary vasoconstrictor) therapy continued for several days but then slowed such that she could be discharged. However, four weeks later, she was continuing to use ten pads per day and felt weak. She developed a sore mouth and gums, ecchymosis (bruises), and petechiae (capillary micro-hemorrhages) of the upper and lower extremities. She was readmitted to the outlying hospital, received two units of blood, and was discharged after the bleeding stopped for four days. Bleeding then recurred and was quite extensive. She also complained of severe occipital (posterior skull) headaches and arrangements for admission to MCGH were made. On admission, the patient had the sudden onset of left upper arm tingling, numbness, and weakness. Her tongue "felt thick" and speaking was difficult. Her face felt as if it had been "shot full of Novocaine". Her past history revealed an episode of Graves' disease (thyroid inflammatory disease) treated with drugs for several months and then subtotal thyroidectomy. She required radioactive iodine therapy later for recurrent Graves' disease. Physical examination revealed some exophthalmos (bulging prominence of the eyes often seen with thyroid disease). Vital signs were normal. Petechiae (small punctate skin hemorrhages) were present on the tongue and extremities. Ecchymosis (bruises) were present on the legs. Liver and spleen were not palpable. Initial diagnosis was possible diuretic drug-induced thrombocytopenic purpura (bruising and petechiae related to low platelet count clotting factor) or possible idiopathic (unknown etiology) thrombocytopenic purpura. Her early hospital course revealed three spells of reported numbness and tingling of the left arm that were not observed. Prednisone (steroid) therapy was started. About one week following admission she had the sudden onset of expressive dysphasia (difficulty speaking—mixed up "word salad"), staring, drooling, and dysphagia (difficulty swallowing) lasting about ten minutes, with slurred speech going on for two hours, followed by sleepiness. A neurologic consultation was obtained from Dr. De Oliviera who described her as alert, having expressive dysphasia and dysnomia, dysgraphia, (difficulty repeating names and recognizing letters written on her skin with a finger), and verbal perseveration (repeating phrases and words). She followed commands. There was equivocal left-sided weakness, but the deep tendon reflexes were equal and no pathological reflexes were present. Sensory examination was normal. A diagnosis of ischemia in the distribution of the right middle cerebral artery was made. Electroencephalogram (EEG) was abnormal showing focal right hemisphere as well as multifocal and generalized dysfunction of an acute nature. The following day she had definite left-sided weakness and was more obtunded and was observed to have Jacksonian (focal) seizures. Prednisone dosage was doubled. 24 hours later she was febrile to 101°. There was left hemiparesis (paralysis), left lower facial flattening, and she was now aphasic (unable to speak) as well as being confused, having a poor response to commands, and obvious difficulty swallowing. She became comatose. She was treated with high-dose prednisone as well as heparin, low molecular weight dextran (blood volume expander), Imuran (immune system stimulator), and antibiotics. Over the next five days she had changing levels of consciousness but was mostly comatose. Blood was oozing from her nose, mouth, nasogastric tube, vagina, and rectum. Grand mal (major diffuse) and Jacksonian seizures were occurring. Except for a temperature elevation to 103°, vital signs remained stable; lungs were clear, heart tones were normal, and bowel sounds were normal. Increasing petechiae and ecchymosis were present. Less than 24 hours after this rapid deterioration, the patient died. Laboratory values of interest were an anemia down to 7.6 g of hemoglobin (normal 12-16), platelet counts from 7,000 – 34,000 (normal 150,000-250,000). Reticulocyte (red blood cell precursors) counts were as high as 36 percent (normal <2 percent). LE (Lupus) antinuclear factor was negative. Complement (immune factor) was normal. Bleeding time was 7 min., clotting time 8.5 min., Protime 14.5 sec., Factor V 67 percent, fibrinogen 276. (All quite normal clotting factors). Blood smear consisted mostly of schistocytes (red blood cells that are broken and partially destroyed). Bone marrow had normal megakaryocytes (platelet precursors). **Pathologic diagnosis of Case Number Two:** This young patient died of Thrombotic Thrombocytopenic Purpura (TTP). The clinical diagnosis usually is confirmed by the pathological finding of widespread hyaline (waxey) occlusion of terminal arterioles and capillaries accompanied by vascular lesions at the arteriolar-capillary junction often involving heart, brain, kidneys, pancreas, and adrenal glands. It can occur from infancy to the elderly but peaks in the third decade, which is compatible with our patient. Hemorrhagic and neurologic manifestations are the most frequent presenting complaints and findings. The neurologic manifestations are due to small vessel involvement in the gray matter of the brain and brainstem. The fragmented red blood cells are probably related to a microangiopathy (inflamed, diseased small blood vessels) that leads to a hemolytic (red-cell destroying) anemia and to the markedly elevated reticulocyte counts.

Comments: In retrospect, the first case should have been diagnosed clinically with a high degree of suspicion for pulmonary emboli and possibly earlier institution of anticoagulation. Identifying the presence of an atrial septal defect would have been very problematic in the 1960s prior to the availability of echocardiography. The thrombotic effect of sickle cell disease may have been a significant contributor to her demise.

The second case was a nightmare for me. I spent most of her hospitalization at her bedside, trying to "put out the fires" that kept popping-up. Just when it would seem that she was stabilizing, a new and fresh deterioration occurred, for which I had few answers. Today, TTP remains a life-threatening illness of serious proportions, but newer treatment modalities such as plasmapheresis (plasma "cleansing" by machines) have markedly reduced the death rate and complications of this illness. I am still eternally grateful to Dr. De Oliviera of neurology, who spent almost as much time with this patient as I did, and was able to describe the microneurologic lesions that were occurring as part of the clinical syndrome. It probably was one of the most profound faculty teaching relationships I had during my residency.

After three years as a medical resident it was time to move on again. The following chapter will describe that journey.

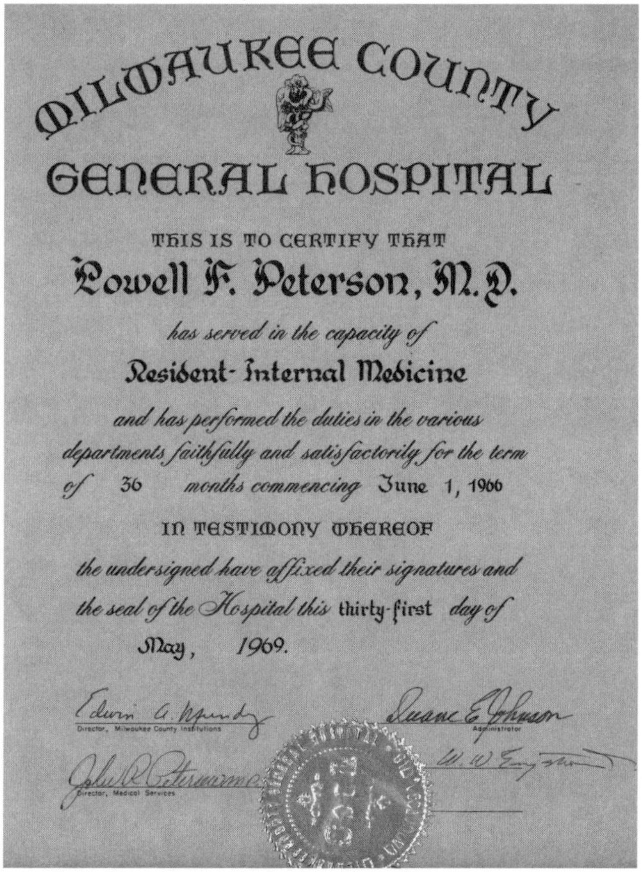

MILWAUKEE COUNTY
GENERAL HOSPITAL

THIS IS TO CERTIFY THAT

Powell F. Peterson, M.D.

has served in the capacity of

Resident- Internal Medicine

and has performed the duties in the various departments faithfully and satisfactorily for the term of 36 *months commencing* June 1, 1966

IN TESTIMONY WHEREOF

the undersigned have affixed their signatures and the seal of the Hospital this thirty-first *day of* May, 1969.

Director, Milwaukee County Institutions

Administrator

Director, Medical Services

Chapter Ten

CARDIOLOGY FELLOWSHIP

(1969-1970)

In July of 1969, following three years of an internal medicine residency program, I began my cardiology training at Milwaukee County General Hospital (MCGH). I was very fortunate, through a quirk of luck, to be accepted into this fellowship program. There were only two fellowship positions in cardiology and both were taken. Without any forewarning, one of the accepted fellows suddenly resigned from the program before he even started. I learned later that he was from Panama, where a political revolution was underway, and he felt obligated to return home to help protect and stabilize his family. The chief of cardiology at MCGH was livid, as he was left without a second fellow, which reflected negatively on him and his program. One of my colleagues discovered this turn of events and suggested that if I was interested, I should quickly go down to the cardiology office and apply for the position, which I did. Up until this point, I thought I would focus on internal medicine and probably work in a multi-specialty clinic, but when I heard the news that I might have a shot at this fellowship, I found myself suddenly anxious to apply. This turn of events jolted my memory back to an afternoon during my residency—an experience that should have tipped me off that I might want to pursue cardiology. That day, an assistant professor of cardiology, Dr. Mike Keelan, took me to the radiology suite to observe him place a temporary pacemaker catheter into the right ventricle of a patient's heart. The X-ray machine was archaic by today's standards and required fluoroscopic viewing through a green-colored glass port about the size of a small dinner plate. I watched as Dr. Keelan passed the catheter and positioned it, but in spite of restoring a paced cardiac rhythm, electromechanical dissociation (electrical pacing without muscular contraction response) occurred, with the heart unable to maintain cardiac output (blood forward flow) and blood pressure. The patient was pronounced dead on the X-ray table. By this time in my medical training I had seen many patients die and it no longer shocked me. As the doctor began to remove the now useless pacing wire, he paused to look at me and asked, "Would you like to try manipulating the wire into the heart?" It may seem somewhat ghoulish to a layperson, but as a medical resident, I didn't hesitate. Doctor Keelan stepped aside and for the next few minutes I practiced guiding the catheter into position. It was my first direct experience with the human heart of a patient, and I admit that it fascinated me beyond all expectation. Although I have manipulated catheters into all chambers of the heart and into the coronary arteries over the ensuing 40 years, I still remember the excitement I felt with that first attempt. That energized feeling never left me.

I was thrilled when I was accepted as the second cardiac fellow and therefore, the uncertainty I had felt about my career direction was markedly diminished. The other cardiology fellow, Dr. Donald Tresch, was from the University of Wisconsin and was a very intelligent, friendly, hard-working individual. We had an excellent working relationship throughout the next year. I felt very fortunate that I would be taught by a vast array of excellent cardiologists, each with their own expertise, during this fellowship year.

Cardiac catheterization and coronary arteriography (passing catheters into the heart and visualizing the heart and blood vessels with the injection of radio-opaque solution) were relatively new to the medical world at the time I started my fellowship. The initial reports of success with this procedure came from Dr. Mason Sones' laboratory at the Cleveland Clinic in the early 1960s. Soon after, catheterization laboratories blossomed throughout the country and Milwaukee became a hotbed of competition for cases at multiple hospitals. Technological advances in X-ray equipment were necessary to guarantee that adequate diagnostic studies of the heart and coronary arteries could be achieved and recorded on 35mm movie film in real time. Powerful X-ray generators and sophisticated image intensifiers became available as several large industrial companies in this country and in Europe and Asia competed for the burgeoning market. Of course, this was all driven by the equally new cardiac surgery programs initiated in the 1960s in Cleveland, Minneapolis, Milwaukee, the Mayo Clinic, and others from coast to coast, demonstrating the feasibility of bypassing obstructed coronary arteries with vein grafts.

An active cardiac catheterization laboratory was up and running at MCGH prior to my entering the fellowship, and to my great benefit, the staff physicians in cardiology were adept in coronary arteriography. In the next year I would carry out diagnostic cardiac catheterization and coronary arteriography studies on over 100 patients. My mentors taught me the innovative Sones technique, passing catheters through arm vessels under X-ray fluoroscopic control into the heart and coronary arteries. Years later, sheaths were developed for entering the femoral artery and vein (at the groin crease) and this eventually became the catheterization procedure of choice.

Just as with cardiac catheterization, pacemaker therapy for complete heart block (blocked transmission of the heart's electrical impulses to cause muscular contraction), or for periods of asystole (complete absence of electrical impulses), was also in its infancy. The first pacemaker I saw during medical school was an external pacemaker with the generator roughly the size of a large TV console connected by wires to electrodes on a rubber strap around the chest to deliver shocks to the heart through the chest wall. By the time I started my internship, implantable pacemakers were installed by a surgeon who would perform a thoracotomy (opening the chest), sewing the electrode wires directly onto the heart. The pacemaker generators, placed under the skin on the chest wall, were at least the size of hockey pucks and weighed about a pound each. The life expectancy of the battery units was 18 months. The generators worked at a fixed rate even if there were occasional native heartbeats, a potentially dangerous situation. The alternative however, was syncope (black outs) or sudden death. By the late 1960s, the electrode catheters could be passed through veins to the heart without opening the chest. Thanks to technological advancements, bit-by-bit over the next several years, the paced heart rate became adjustable, the pacemaker worked on demand rather than at a fixed rate, lithium batteries extended the life of the pacemaker, and transistors and microprocessors improved the

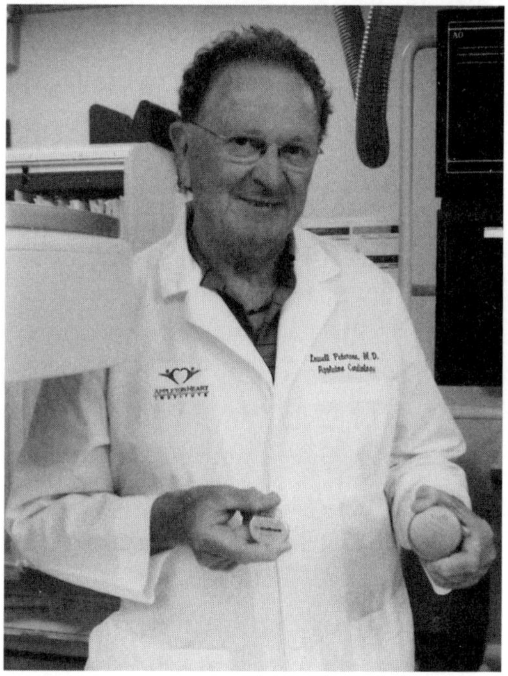

Demonstrating the difference in size of Pacemakers (since the year 2000, left - back in 1970, right)

electronics. Today, pacemakers are about the size of two 50-cent pieces stacked on top of each other and last up to six years before a change is necessary. I was taught in my fellowship how to place the electrode wires through the external jugular (superficial neck vein), cephalic (vein near the shoulder), or the subclavian (vein under the clavicle), and how to create a pocket under the skin of the chest for the generator without resorting to thoracotomy or general anesthesia.

With excellent mentors I quickly learned to insert pacemakers without difficulty. One of my earliest cases, however, did present a problem after the pacer insertion was completed and the patient was transferred to the intensive care unit on the top floor of the hospital. Shortly after arriving there, the nurses reported the pacemaker stopped pacing and the patient was periodically blacking out. I assumed the electrode wire had become dislodged and lost contact with the heart. The patient was quickly taken back to the X-ray suite, and although the pacemaker was working well at that point, I opened the incision and repositioned the electrode wire, and the patient again returned to the intensive care unit. In less than 15 minutes, the nurses called again with the same message and the patient was brought back to the cardiology X-ray suite again. It was noted the pacemaker was functioning appropriately, and the patient was observed for a period of time without re-opening the pocket or manipulating the electrode wires, and then transferred back to the ICU. I soon received another call noting a malfunction. At this point I became suspicious that the problem wasn't originating in the pacemaker, but in the ICU. Was something interfering with the electromechanical function of the pacemaker? I didn't know, but I moved the patient to a regular medical ward with a portable monitor and there were no further difficulties. The patient was discharged after a few days. I notified the biomedical personnel of the hospital who immediately initiated an investigation of the ICU for any stray voltage problems. They determined that a TV-VHF or UHF transmitter tower on the top of a downtown Milwaukee hotel was beaming its signal directly toward the upper floors of the hospital, and it was likely this signal was shutting down the electronic function of the pacemaker. After that, a separate cardiology ICU was established on a lower floor of the hospital and I never had this problem again.

One of the most frightening pacemaker generator change cases I experienced was on a patient who was totally dependent on the pacemaker for initiating his heartbeats. As I extracted the previously implanted pacing wire from the old (to be replaced) generator, the wire stripped and the outer plastic coating tore off. After a few moments of terror with no heart beat (an "Oh, S____" moment) I was able to connect a temporary pacemaker to a single hair-thin strand of wire visible in the frayed wire and achieved pacing, saving the patient's life. I quickly inserted a new permanent wire into the heart and attached the new generator to it. It then became a "whew!" moment. I was very thankful for how well I had been trained to understand predicaments such as this and improvise a solution.

In 1967, prior to my fellowship year, I attended an international cardiology conference in San Francisco, which probably influenced my interest in cardiology as well. The highlight of the convention was a presentation by Dr. Christiaan Barnard, who had just performed the first heart transplantation procedure in South Africa. In spite of the usual controversy in the medical community over something new and unique, the extraordinary enthusiasm by the public for this life-salvage procedure, gave hope to many patients where there had been no hope. Soon the procedure was being performed worldwide. Today 2,200 heart transplants are done yearly. I felt fortunate to be present as another milestone in the march to conquer the deadly killer, heart disease, was proclaimed.

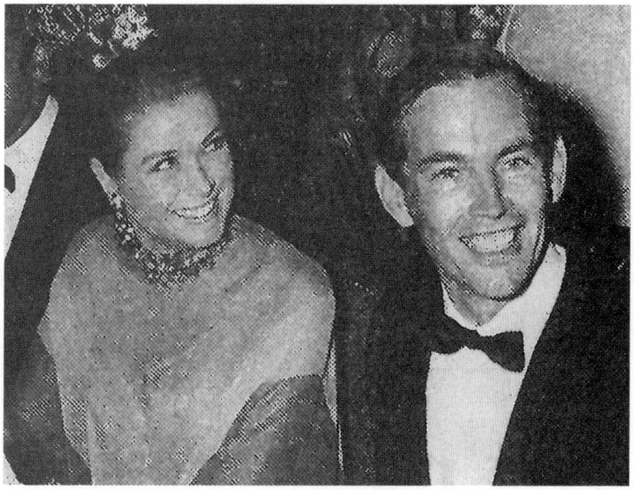

Princess Grace accompanied by Christiaan Barnard

Working in the outpatient clinic each week, I evaluated new patients or patients with chronic cardiology problems referred there for evaluation. It was educational and allowed me to follow patients for a longer period of time. One of my patients was an elegant young black woman who was always well dressed and wore an expensive leather coat. I remember this because her appearance was so unusual compared to our usual poor black, and indigent white, clinic clientele. I looked forward to her appointments not only because she was so striking, but because she always had interesting stories to share and I enjoyed our conversations. Her cardiac condition was rather minor—a prolapse of the mitral valve that caused mild mitral valve regurgitation of blood retrograde from the left ventricle to the left atrium during systole (cardiac contraction). Upon examination, I could hear a very typical systolic cardiac murmur and early systolic click but clinically she had no symptoms.

One Saturday morning near the end of my fellowship year, my wife and I were driving to Rockford, Illinois, where I had a recruiting interview. As we passed through southern Wisconsin we were listening to WTMJ radio, when suddenly, a news bulletin came over the radio stating that the First Wisconsin National Bank in downtown Milwaukee had just been held up at gunpoint by an attractive black woman in high heels and a long, brown leather coat. She handed the teller a note demanding money while brandishing a silver-plated revolver. She placed the folded money in her Gucci purse, turned around and walked out. I about drove off the road. I turned to my wife and said, "That's a patient of mine!" Later news bulletins noted that she was quickly apprehended and was being booked at police headquarters. I honestly did not expect that I would ever see her back in the clinic, but a few weeks later, presumably out on bail, she walked into my clinic for her regular appointment. I asked her, "What in the world ever prompted you to do such a thing?" She didn't miss a beat, answering with a matter-of-fact tone, "I don't know. It just seemed to be the thing to do at the time." I didn't ask any other questions. I was nearing the end of my fellowship so I did not give her a follow-up appointment. I suggested that she re-register in the clinic at a future date if she felt a need to be seen. I gave her a hug and we parted. I'd had another lesson in "street-smarts".

As for my interview in Rockford, it did not go very well. The clinic and hospital I interviewed with really had no concept of how to start a cardiology or cardiac surgery program. There was only one internist on the staff who was interested in cardiology, and he had limited knowledge of the rapidly advancing sphere of cardiology. I was familiar with their general surgeon who trained at MCGH and rated him somewhat below average in his talents. He said that he was going to do the cardiac surgery and that his general surgery training was adequate preparation for taking on this new endeavor. I felt that his attitude and the entire attitude of this clinic and hospital were unrealistic. A competing hospital had started a cardiac surgery program and did have a trained cardiologist and cardiac surgeon, which was an improvement, but I felt this program was in its infancy and there really was no place for me.

Fortunately for me, one day near the end of my fellowship, I was introduced to Dr. Tom Ryan, a former internal medicine resident and chief resident at MCGH who was now practicing as an internist in Appleton, Wisconsin. Tom was on a recruiting mission to his alma mater residency, looking for internists or subspecialists who might be interested in joining his group. He was especially interested in recruiting a trained cardiologist because Appleton Memorial Hospital was aggressively developing a cardiac catheterization laboratory that would be completed and functional within two months after I finished my fellowship. It sounded like it could be a great fit, so I agreed to take a road trip north and check it out.

Before that, however, I made arrangements for an interview at the Marshfield Clinic in Marshfield, Wisconsin, my wife's hometown. Although her parents had both passed away, she continued to own and maintain their home. Our weekend visit to Marshfield was very pleasant and we were treated well with tours of the hospital and clinic, dinner at the country club, and an opportunity for me to make rounds on cardiology and cardiac surgery patients. I also attended a cardiology conference as a guest of the senior cardiologist, Dr. Dean Emanuel.

My subsequent visit to Appleton was also very cordial and, again, we were entertained and given the opportunity to assess the program that included a consultation service at several outlying hospitals within a 60-mile radius. Tom Ryan's associates, Dr. Gene Danford and Dr. John Mielke, were very aggressive internists and well acclimated to subspecialty work. Dr. Mielke was a driving force behind the development of the catheterization laboratory and was undergoing additional cardiology training at St. Luke's Hospital in Milwaukee. It seemed to me that my potential colleagues wanted to build a cardiology center that could rival the best. I wanted in. I agreed to commit myself as the fourth member of the Internal Medicine Associates. I was invited to dessert at Dr. Danford's house after a group dinner with our wives at a nice restaurant. During the conversation I was asked what I would require for a salary. I was offered around $15,000 a year at Marshfield, but I had read ads in the *New England Journal of Medicine* listing starting salaries for internists as $22,000 a year. So, that's what I asked for, rather sheepishly I might add. Everyone looked at each other in a rather dumbfounded manner, which I could not interpret. I found out later they had expected me to ask for a much higher remuneration as a cardiologist, rather than a salary as a general internist. They all quickly recovered their composure and immediately agreed to my request and arranged to have their business manager, Terry Woodford, draw up a contract.

I was elated with this turn of events but I really was very sad when I had to sit down and write Dr. Emanuel a letter stating that I had decided to go to Appleton rather than to Marshfield. Forty years later I attended an event at the Laird Center for Medical Research at the Marshfield Clinic and talked with Dr. Emanuel. I told him that each time I visited Marshfield I wondered if I made a mistake by choosing to practice in Appleton. In his gentlemanly fashion, he stated, "No Lowell, you did not." My cordial relationship with many of the staff members there continues to this day.

The truth is, I could have stayed for another year of cardiology fellowship and become familiar with other new and emerging techniques, such as echocardiography, a clinical evaluation tool that studies the heart via reflected ultrasound waves. One more year would also have afforded me the opportunity to become board certified in cardiology in addition to my certification by the American Board of Internal Medicine. At the time, these facts still didn't trump my gut feeling that it was time to move on. Or, as my chief of cardiology, Dr. Lange, put it when I asked his advice, "I think it is time for you to go to work." His words provided me with the validation I needed. I was emotionally devastated when he died of pancreatic cancer less than two years later.

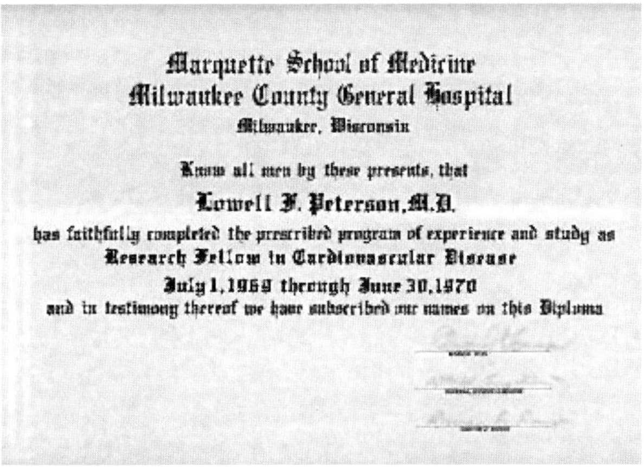
Marquette School of Medicine
Milwaukee County General Hospital
Milwaukee, Wisconsin
Know all men by these presents, that
Lowell F. Peterson, M.D.
has faithfully completed the prescribed program of experience and study as
Research Fellow in Cardiovascular Disease
July 1, 1969 through June 30, 1970
and in testimony thereof we have subscribed our names on this Diploma

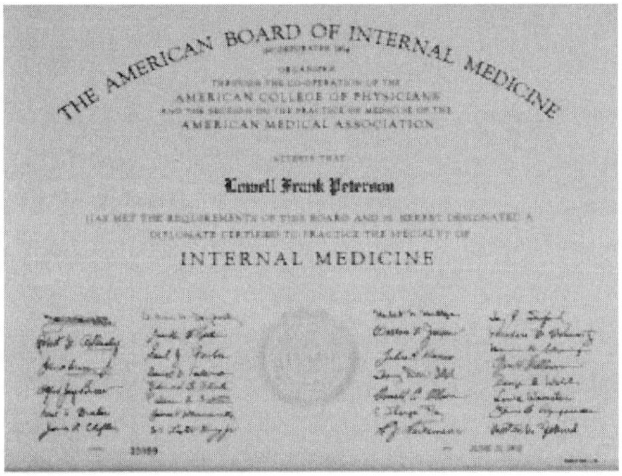
THE AMERICAN BOARD OF INTERNAL MEDICINE
ORGANIZED
THROUGH THE CO-OPERATION OF THE
AMERICAN COLLEGE OF PHYSICIANS
AND THE SECTION ON THE PRACTICE OF MEDICINE OF THE
AMERICAN MEDICAL ASSOCIATION
ATTESTS THAT
Lowell Frank Peterson
HAS MET THE REQUIREMENTS OF THIS BOARD AND IS HEREBY DESIGNATED A
DIPLOMATE CERTIFIED TO PRACTICE THE SPECIALTY OF
INTERNAL MEDICINE

So, after four years in Milwaukee, my wife and I headed up Highway 41 to Appleton, very much aware that we were making a major life decision that would shape our family's future. I had no idea how I would fare, moving from an academic training program into private practice, but I knew it was time to try.

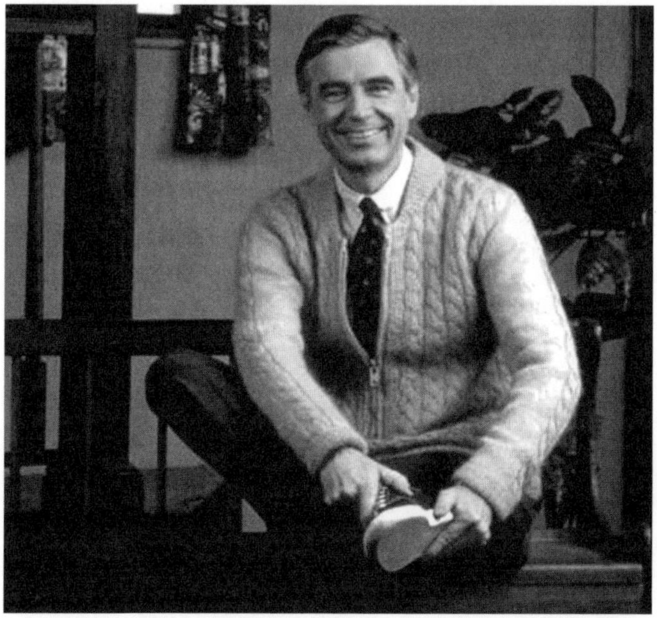

"When you combine your own intuition with a sensitivity to other people's feelings and moods, you may be close to the origins of valuable human attributes such as generosity, altruism, compassion, sympathy, and empathy."

—Fred Rogers
The World According to Mr. Rogers
"Important Things to Remember"
Hyperion, 77 W. 66th Street
New York, NY 10023-6298
www.hyperionbooks.com

Chapter Eleven

THE APPLETON ADVENTURE BEGINS

(1970-1980)

After choosing to take the job offer in Appleton, my wife, Mary, and I started house hunting. We had three children less than seven years of age and we needed to find a house big enough for our new beginning and—with luck—for the many years to come. We had never had to reach consensus on anything this momentous, and the decision to take on a mortgage was especially daunting after living on a miniscule resident's salary supplemented by the G. I. Bill. Fortunately, my wife found a suitable, newly-constructed house on Beechwood Court very near my new office in Doctor's Park, and about five minutes from Appleton Memorial Hospital. As I was wrapping up loose ends in Milwaukee, Mary signed the contract and made a down payment. Our mortgage was arranged through the First National Bank, facilitated by the financial advisor of my new medical corporation, Terry Woodford, and the attorney of his choice, Peter Nelson. So there we were, taking a new job, buying a new house, and feeling the same way all adults do when they suddenly realize they've reached responsible adulthood: anxious, confused, and excited.

As we were emptying boxes and arranging furniture in our new home, Dr. John Mielke drove up in his beat-up, nearly antique, Ford, and welcomed us to the city. Then he asked me if I was ready to go to work. I said, "Of course." He said, Dr. Simon Cherkasky had requested a consultation on a patient at St. Elizabeth's Hospital. I accepted the challenge and was off and running, utilizing my medical knowledge for the first time in a fee-for-service setting. It was not anything earth shattering in terms of medicine, but it gave me an unforgettable ego boost as I launched my career. Very soon, consultation requests for difficult medical and cardiac problems began to come in from other general practice physicians and internists, as well as general surgeons and specialty surgeons. Some may have simply been curious to test the new guy on the block, but in most cases the doctor requested I take over the entire management of the case. Many of these patients were very difficult to diagnose and treat because they had multiple disease processes, had grown old right along with their doctors, and were a bit skeptical about trusting their care to someone new. My associates, Drs. Danford, Mielke, and Ryan were very talented and I felt the trust conferred on me by the referring physicians and their patients was also a reflection of the respect the community afforded them.

I quickly became acquainted with Appleton Memorial Hospital, (the location of the new cardiovascular laboratory), and also with its first-class intensive care unit (ICU). I also visited St. Elizabeth's hospital daily and became equally familiar with its facilities.

After a short two-week respite of day-to-day medicine and cardiology practice and a period of familiarization with the hospitals and the community, my associates felt I was ready to go it alone with night and weekend-call. I was nervous and concerned about assuming this lonely, but challenging endeavor. Fortunately, Dr. Tom Ryan agreed to mentor me and reassured me that he would be available by telephone for any questions or concerns. Little did I know, that on my very first night on-call, on a weekend, I would be faced with one of the most horrendous cardiology problems I would ever encounter. I received a call from one of the outlying hospitals that a physician from a small community had just entered their hospital with an acute myocardial infarction (heart attack) and his colleague, the attending physician, wanted—no, insisted—on transferring the patient to my care at Appleton Memorial Hospital. I quickly checked with Dr. Ryan as to the advisability of immediate transfer as opposed to stabilizing the patient in the local hospital. Following his advice, I soon learned that it is best to rapidly stabilize the patient and then quickly transfer, especially if the patient has worrisome vital signs and unrelieved pain. Upon arrival at Appleton Memorial Hospital, the doctor-patient was anything but stable. Vital signs were fluctuating wildly and multiple intravenous drugs were required to stabilize the blood pressure, heart rate, and lung congestion as well as suppress cardiac rhythm abnormalities. He was cool, clammy, and diaphoretic—all signs of shock. Intravenous morphine was given in an attempt to control chest pain as well as to allay anxiety, but in spite of this, the patient continued to have periodic episodes of accelerated, severe chest pain throughout the night. The vital sign stabilization and pain control efforts were like trying to juggle six balls with one hand because of the rapidly changing condition of the patient. I remained at the patient's bedside in the intensive care unit throughout the night and made periodic calls to Dr. Ryan for his advice and reassurance. The patient's family was kept informed of his condition and they remained at his bedside as well. In spite of my valiant efforts, the patient had one last extremely excruciating chest pain that made him scream, as he died. The autopsy confirmed my suspicion that each of the accelerated episodes of chest pain in spite of vigorous morphine therapy was related to progressive dissection of blood into the severely damaged myocardium (heart muscle), softened by the loss of coronary circulation, with the final result being cardiac rupture and cardiac tamponade (blood filling the pericardial sac and compressing the heart). In future years, with increasing cardiac surgical capabilities, this patient might have survived with open-heart surgery and infarctectomy (removal of the damaged heart muscle) with placement of a patch and a sutured repair. But even with these heroics, the mortality rate would be extremely high. Suturing in the soft, damaged muscle, is like placing stitches in wet tissue paper. This case left me with mixed emotions. Although I did everything I could possibly do for the patient, I was left with a sense of failure because I lost the patient. It would not be the last time I would experience these deep feelings. The practice of medicine walks a fine line between life and death, especially in the ICU—a narrow path too frequently traveled.

In the late 1960s my associates established a remote monitoring system for patients in several surrounding community hospitals using a dedicated telephone line. With this system the ICU nurses were able to visualize a patient's cardiac rhythm on monitors in the intensive care unit at St. Elizabeth's Hospital. This was cutting edge technology, particularly for rural hospitals. Only one other telephone network of this type (in Oklahoma) was being utilized anywhere in the country. One of the very first patients I observed on this remote monitoring system was a man who showed evidence of complete heart block (failure to propagate electrical impulses to the heart muscle). He was dropping heartbeats, had a heart rate of 30 beats per minute, and sometimes experienced long pauses without a heartbeat which caused loss of consciousness. I quickly called the attending physician at the remote hospital and arranged for immediate ambulance transfer to Appleton. Upon his arrival the patient was taken directly to the X-ray department where I placed a temporary pacemaker wire into his heart. His heart block did not subside spontaneously and, therefore, I installed a permanent pacemaker a couple of days later. He lived, and worked many more symptom-free years on his farm, and I performed several pacemaker generator changes for him in the ensuing years.

Our group worked tirelessly to establish our reputation in Appleton and beyond. We had a presence at the hospital in Kaukauna, Wisconsin, a few miles to the east of Appleton, where Dr. Ryan provided the primary consultative service. While covering for Dr. Ryan, or when I was on-call on nights or weekends, I received many calls in the middle of the night from anxious Kaukauna general practitioners concerning patients with chest pain or heart failure, requesting I come to see the patient. I never refused, but many times I felt quite sure, even before I arrived, that the patient would require transfer to the ICU, either at Appleton Memorial or St. Elizabeth's. I remember making one of these runs to the Kaukauna Hospital at three in the morning on glare-ice roads only to confirm that the patient needed to be transferred to Appleton. Still, it was important for me to confirm in person that this was the right course of action, and I also knew that meeting the specialist solidified for the family and the patient that their doctor was in charge and was doing the best thing he could for them. The clinic in Kaukauna continues to thrive but the hospital closed several years ago.

Our group also consulted in several other outlying hospitals within 60 miles of Appleton, including Waupaca, New London, Clintonville, Shawano, Chilton, and Berlin. In later years, additional communities were added. Another unique service provided to the rural hospitals was the ability to transmit an entire electrocardiogram (EKG) by telephone directly to our office. This required personnel on both ends of the phone line to establish the connection and proceed with the sending and receiving. When a call was received at night to transmit an EKG, it required the doctor on-call to get up, go to the office, arrange for the transmission, receive the tracings, interpret the tracings, and call the hospital back with the report. Cumbersome as it was, it worked. Because of this service, lives were saved. In 1978 we introduced a computer into the AMH-ICU that could interpret EKGs, but during daytime hours these were all reviewed by an EKG-qualified internist or cardiologist for accuracy. Any EKG requiring a stat over-read at night was sent to our home by taxi or police car. Thank God, with improved computers and software, things have changed since those days, but I must say, that during that early pioneering period, we did provide a tremendous service to a good share of northeastern Wisconsin.

I began my personal outreach service in 1970 at the Calumet Memorial Hospital in Chilton, Wisconsin, about 50 miles from Appleton. In those days of the hippie era, I let my hair grow quite long and I had a bushy mustache. My wife enjoyed picking out clothes for me. I bought dapper suits and sport coats in Milwaukee assisted by a young entrepreneur/salesman, Steve Schroeder, who would eventually own his upscale store, Roger-Stevens, at the Pfister Hotel on E. Wisconsin Avenue. I don't think the nurses at the Chilton Hospital ever saw anything quite like me. Most of their local general practitioners dressed very casually or with their only two-piece or three-piece Sunday suit. The nurses often would joke that they could not wait for my next weekly visit to see what kind of loud tie and extravagant sport coat I would be wearing.

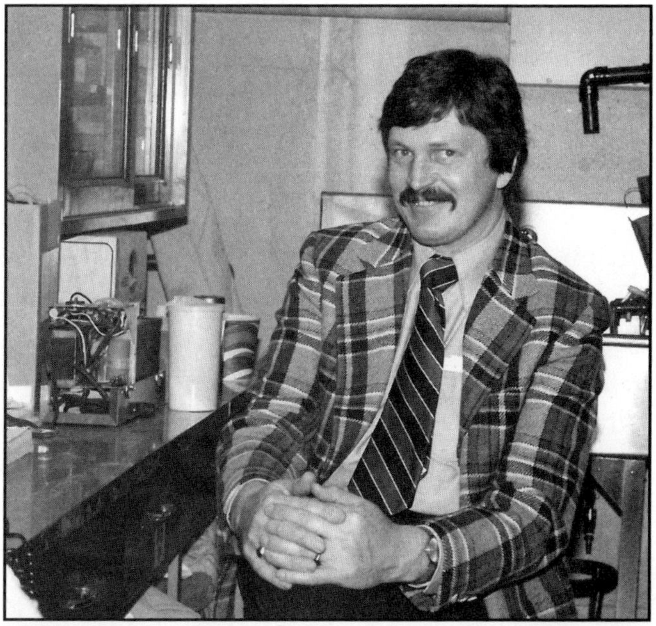

Occasionally, patients also made a fuss about my appearance. One farmer who was a patient at AMH would accost me each morning while I was making rounds and tell me to get a haircut. He also noted that, back on the farm, he cut the hair of his boys and he would never tolerate them looking like me. After several days of this useless irritation I had had enough. I told him, "Look, I know you don't like my long hair, but it's what's inside the head that counts, not what's outside." I guess he thought about that and accepted it. He never mentioned the subject again.

In the early 1970s, Dr. Ryan requested to be relieved of his consultative services at Riverside Hospital in Waupaca, Wisconsin, and confine his practice to the Appleton hospitals and the Kaukauna Hospital. My group asked me if I would take over the Waupaca hospital service. I was somewhat reluctant to do this because I grew up near Waupaca and I was sure I would see patients that had known me from when I was a little boy—or worse—when I was a mischievous adolescent or teen. Nevertheless, I agreed to give it a try and was very pleased to be treated as a local boy who made good and had come home to serve his community. One of my nurses noted recently, "You walk on water out there; they love you." I was sure that any doctor who chose to dedicate time and career to this small community would hear the same compliment. Nevertheless, I took the hyperbole to heart and my love for the nurses, doctors, and patients, was reciprocal. Our pleasant and wonderful relationship would go on for more than 38 years until my retirement. Many of the older physicians working in that community hospital knew me from my college and medical school days. Drs. Sam Salan, Marshall Boudry, John Steiner, Kenneth Haman, Lloyd Maasch, and Numeriano Hollero, along with the multiple specialty doctors, particularly, Dr. Fred Smith, and Dr. Joe Skibba, were more than kind in providing me with hands-on experience in those college and med school years. As I entered medical practice, these relationships to the community helped me build my practice in Appleton as well as in Waupaca. Dr. Jerry Salan joined his father in practice in the late '60s, becoming the nidus for establishment of the ever-expanding Waupaca Family Medicine Clinic in years to come. Jerry and I were quite close in age and because he was also a local Waupaca boy, we established very strong ties professionally.

On one occasion in the early 1970s our group decided that the remote rural hospitals should receive two visits per week rather than just one so that we could better follow the patients' progress. One person would be assigned to make this second visit at all of the hospitals on Friday because we did not have the manpower to send each physician out twice per week. Despite our good intentions, this was one of the most stressful undertakings we initiated. I remember being called to Theda Clark Hospital in the early morning hours of a Friday to see a patient in the intensive care unit, which took a couple of hours. I then went home, shaved, showered, and returned to make my rounds on patients at both Appleton hospitals before going back to Theda Clark Hospital to check on the patient in the ICU. Afterward, I drove east to Chilton to follow-up with patients seen earlier in the week, see new consults, and read EKGs. I then drove west to New London, Clintonville, and Waupaca, carrying out the same functions at each stop. My food for the day was a hamburger and malted milk purchased at the DQ in Clintonville. There was no

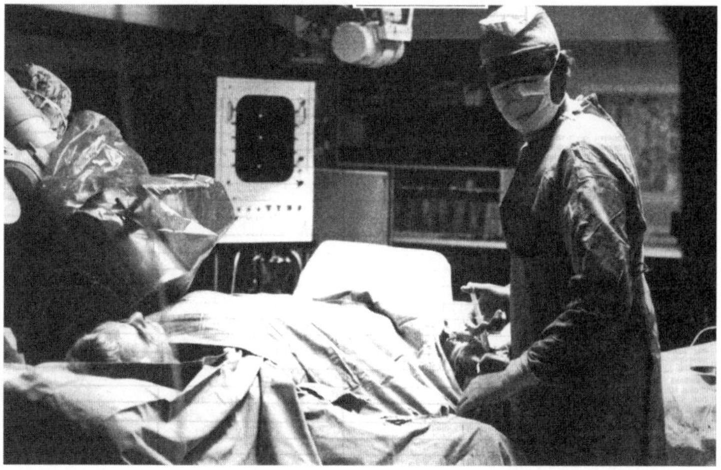

drink holder in my 1966 Mustang, so I attempted to hold the shake with my feet on the floor as I drove to Waupaca. Of course, it tipped and spilled all over the floor-mat, which resulted in a flurry of blue words. I finally arrived home about 9 p.m. after driving about 250 miles and working for 18 hours straight. No matter how much our group wanted to enhance our services to the rural communities, this type of workday was unsustainable. Fortunately, it did not take us long to see the errors of our ways and we unanimously agreed to cancel this program. I should have surmised, however, that there were an awful lot of 18-hour workdays ahead of me.

Although everyone in the group essentially worked as an internist while on-call, the value of our group lay with our experience as specialists. And, with the opening of the cardiovascular laboratory in August 1970, Dr. Mielke and I took our first steps toward making cardiology a sentinel feature of the group. We performed our first cardiac catheterization studies on patients referred by Dr. Tom Loescher, a local general practitioner. Jean Lehndorf, RN, was the head nurse in the laboratory and was instrumental in helping us get the program underway and running smoothly. She would eventually become my personal nurse, working closely with me, both in Appleton and Waupaca, for more than 30 years prior to her retirement. I believe Dr. Mielke and I each performed 100-150 catheterization studies that first year with the patients requiring cardiac surgery for coronary by-pass or valve replacements being transferred to St. Luke's Hospital in Milwaukee to the service of Dr. Derward Lepley, Dr. Dudley Johnson, Dr. Bob Flemma, and Dr. Jim Auer.

In the latter part of that first year of successful Cath. Lab. operation, we became enamored with considering initiating our own cardiac surgery program in Appleton. Dr. Mielke and I both had an excellent relationship with the heart surgeons at St. Luke's and we sought their advice. They were very supportive of our efforts and would do almost anything to promote the cause of coronary bypass surgery, which at that time was the target of unrelenting critical attacks. It was not uncommon, for example, to go to national and international cardiology conferences and during a presentation hear booing, hissing, and downright nasty comments thrown at the surgical or invasive cardiology presenters by non-believer physicians and non-invasive cardiologists. Starting a neophyte heart surgery program in a small community hospital in northeastern Wisconsin, therefore, seemed to many as something less idealistic and a bit Quixotic. Members of the local Appleton-Neenah lay community and medical community were also cautiously skeptical, and a few physicians made no secret about their desire for us to fail.

Dr. Hal Harding, a fully-trained cardiovascular surgery fellow, was recruited from the Milwaukee County and St. Luke's program to start our cardiac surgery program with the full blessing of Drs. Lepley and Johnson. After training his technicians and nurses, as well as recruiting professionals from other programs, the day came when the program was launched. We lived by the principle that failure was not in our vocabulary and the cardiology and cardiac surgery team proceeded full speed ahead. The first coronary bypass procedure at Appleton Memorial Hospital was carried out in August 1971. It was also the first coronary bypass procedure carried out in Wisconsin outside of Milwaukee, Marshfield, La Crosse, and Madison. We worked very hard to establish credibility and presented numerous programs for local and rural hospital physicians, touting the benefits of cardiac surgery for their patients. It was our on the road, "dog-and-pony show". Shortly after starting the surgery program Appleton Memorial Hospital chartered two private airplanes to fly our heart program providers to La Crosse for a cardiology conference. Here we would hear reviews of the cardiac catheterization and cardiac surgery experience of the Gunderson Clinic at Lutheran Hospital. Dr. Mason Sones, the pioneer founder of cardiac catheterization at the Cleveland Clinic was the main speaker, summarizing his experience with more than 2,000 cases in the cath. lab. He also presented the results of the Cleveland coronary bypass surgery experience as pioneered in the mid-1960s by Dr. René Favolaro. Our hospital administrator, Jack Shepard, hospital head nurse, Betty Beyer, cath. lab head nurse, Jean Lehndorf, Dr. Mielke, Dr. Harding, myself, and several technicians and nurses made the trip. Dr. Mielke insisted he and I fly in separate airplanes so that if one of the planes crashed our heart program would not crash with it. We came back from the pep-talk speech from Dr. Sones very enthused to be on the cutting edge of cardiology and cardiac surgery, and very certain we were doing the right thing.

From the beginning, we worked non-stop to increase our practice and be recognized as the premier cardiology and cardiovascular surgery program in northeastern Wisconsin. Perhaps as a sign of our success, in the early 1970s, the Upjohn pharmaceutical company approached us about sponsoring an educational workshop in cardiology for physicians in our area. John Mielke and I met with the drug company's rep. over dinner at Marty's restaurant in Kimberly and finalized the deal over a steak tartare. The first workshop was held at Riverview Country Club, in 1972, and was attended by twelve doctors. I eventually took over the planning of these yearly fall events. I involved more drug companies for financing and expanded the number of physician invitees and began to bring in nationally and internationally recognized experts in the field of cardiology as speakers. The meetings moved to the auditorium at Aid Association for Lutherans (now Thrivent) insurance company, and when we outgrew that facility, the meetings moved to the conference ballrooms at the Paper Valley Hotel. Attendance grew to over 250 doctors, nurses, and other health care professionals. The programs continued yearly for 35 years and I am still proud of how I was able to foster this quality educational forum in northeastern Wisconsin. I consider it one of the highlights of my career.

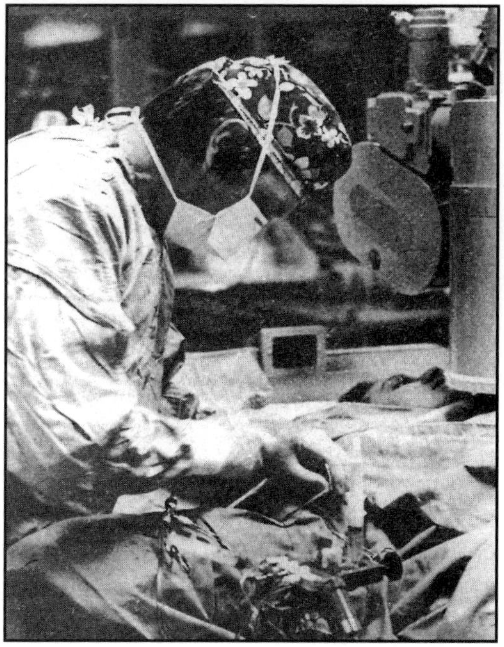

By the mid-1970s, our group's cardiology services were well known and utilized by many hospitals and clinics, including Theda Clark Hospital, in Neenah, Wisconsin. I was already a consultant there and I also hoped to establish a pacemaker service. Some of the referring doctors in this hospital were very cordial to me and did not hesitate to contact me for consultation, pacemaker insertions, and even to refer patients for cardiac catheterization studies at Appleton Memorial Hospital. Nevertheless, an underlying egotistical rivalry existed between Appleton and Neenah, as well as between competing clinics within Neenah itself. I remember an awkward, but amusing instance, when I was sitting at a patient's bedside in a double-bed room at Theda Clark recommending that he come to Appleton for a heart catheterization while at the very same moment a prominent Neenah physician was sitting at the very next bed telling his patient he needed to go to Milwaukee for a heart catheterization. Other times, I heard patients being told their heart problems could be handled without resorting to any newfangled procedures that were offered at Appleton. For some doctors, there was no way they would allow their patients to cross the Fox River to Appleton for anything. The medical staff meetings at Theda Clark were also very confrontational, whether the issue involved the two major clinics, the individual practitioners, a smaller clinic, or those of us who were trying to provide specialty consultation services from Appleton. I spoke at one of these staff meetings about what I had to offer to their community and their hospital in the field of cardiology. I received a cold response. After the meeting, I met one of the local internists about my age whose family had a long medical legacy in this hospital. I pulled him aside and asked why no one seemed excited about the advanced cardiac services I could provide. He looked me straight in the eye and said, "Lowell, you just don't understand the situation." It was a blunt lesson in medical politics, and unfortunately it would not be my last.

Perhaps as a sign of our success, similar cardiology programs within multispecialty groups or as a separate private entity began to appear in neighboring cities. A cardiology fellow with whom I trained at Milwaukee County General Hospital, Dr. Howard Palay, came to Green Bay, Wisconsin, in the mid-1970s, and started his own program. Dr. Ed Scanlon was recruited by Theda Clark Hospital in Neenah, establishing a competing cardiology program which eventually spawned a cardiac surgery program. It was at this point that two opposing points of view emerged: one supported proliferation of programs and one didn't. For my part, I believed having two cardiac surgery programs in such close proximity would only dilute patient volume for each program and would not translate into better services for the community. I felt that if we consolidated our efforts in one program, we had the potential to compete in cardiology and cardiac surgery with anyone in the country. But, it was not to be. It became a battle of egos and trust. The goal of delivering great patient care now would have to go hand-in-glove with petty turf battles and political jockeying among physicians, administrators, and hospital board members. And so it did. Reaching out to other doctors or hospitals to discuss how the programs could work together was a futile exercise and soon enough I became disheartened and finally exhausted by the situation. In fact, the scars of the various squabbles and resentments remain emblazoned on my psyche to this day.

At the time, I remember my cardiology, cardiac surgery, and administrative friends at the Marshfield Clinic assuring me that I could not win this turf battle, and the opposition would prevail, even if it took litigation to accomplish. They were right. Ironically, after several years, the cardiac surgery program at Theda Clark was disbanded, but it then moved even closer to Appleton Medical Center at St. Elizabeth's Hospital, less than two miles away. Go figure!

By the end of the decade of the 1970s, our group had expanded from four members to six with the addition of internist, Dr. Stephen Alt, and gastroenterologist, Dr. Michael Geall, with a goal of forming a multi-specialty clinic. But, it was not to be. In 1980, due to many internal difficulties and inability to recruit quality multi-specialty physicians, a decision was reached to dissolve the group. As president of the organization, I did not relish the thought of being caught in the middle of the controversies that were likely to evolve as the assets of the corporation, right down to the typewriters and paper clips, were distributed. I therefore received approval from the other members to hire our Corporation Counsel to carry out a legal, binding, and equitable distribution. This actually worked very well with a minimum of hard feelings. Suddenly, individual decisions of the members were necessarily made as to what direction their practices were going to take in the future. Dr. Danford and Dr. Geall each elected to establish a single one-man office practice, and Dr. Ryan and Dr. Alt joined in a short-lived dual practice of internal medicine, each eventually going in separate directions.

Prior to the breakup of the Corporation, another cardiologist, Dr. James Cole was recruited to begin practice in Appleton in the spring of 1980. Dr. Mielke and I carried out preliminary talks about forming a cardiology subspecialty practice including Dr. Cole. He agreed to proceed with his commitment and actually found it more palatable to be in a cardiology group rather than a multi-specialty arrangement. Therefore, Dr. Mielke and I, along with our wives, a financial advisor, and an attorney met for what I would call a "Come to Jesus" meeting in the basement rec room of our house, and there we established the groundwork for Appleton Cardiology Associates. We registered as a service corporation (S.C.) with the state of Wisconsin. Because there had been no distribution of assets from the previous Corporation, and because payments would be due to our financial advisor, attorney, and office personnel, as well as to lease office space and provide basic furnishings, Dr. Mielke and I borrowed $10,000 each on our signature to fund the corporation. It is gratifying to know that what started so humbly in the basement of our house, $20,000 in debt, has grown and expanded to a multimillion dollar corporation with 18 cardiologists, several mid-level providers, a supporting staff of nurses, medical assistants, technicians, business office personnel, computer experts, and medical records and chart preparation workers, all managed by a Chief Executive Officer (CEO) and Chief Financial Officer (CFO). It is certainly a gratifying outcome, but one that was not easily achieved.

After our reorganization in 1980 I fought for many years to try and establish a recognizable identity of the cardiology program. Because of my dogged persistence and urging, the multiple loosely connected facets of the cardiac services finally developed a semblance of organization under the banner of the Appleton Heart Institute, but a cohesive entity within its own building structure did not exist for many years. I could not convince the hospital administration to promote the Heart Institute vigorously, or even to put up a sign in front of the hospital designating its existence—this in spite of the fact that the heart program was the major contributor of services financially beneficial to the hospital. Looking back, I have to think there was a paranoia about "the tail wagging the dog" and a fear that promoting the Heart Institute might be offensive to other service providers at the hospital. Eventually, after extensive planning and negotiations, the Appleton Heart Institute opened its own building on the campus of Appleton Medical Center in 2003, bearing its own logo and identity. Finally, the cardiology service had its own brand and its own space where the public could "kick the tires" to see what we had to offer. To this day I am thankful I was able to work within its walls and within the organization for another several years.

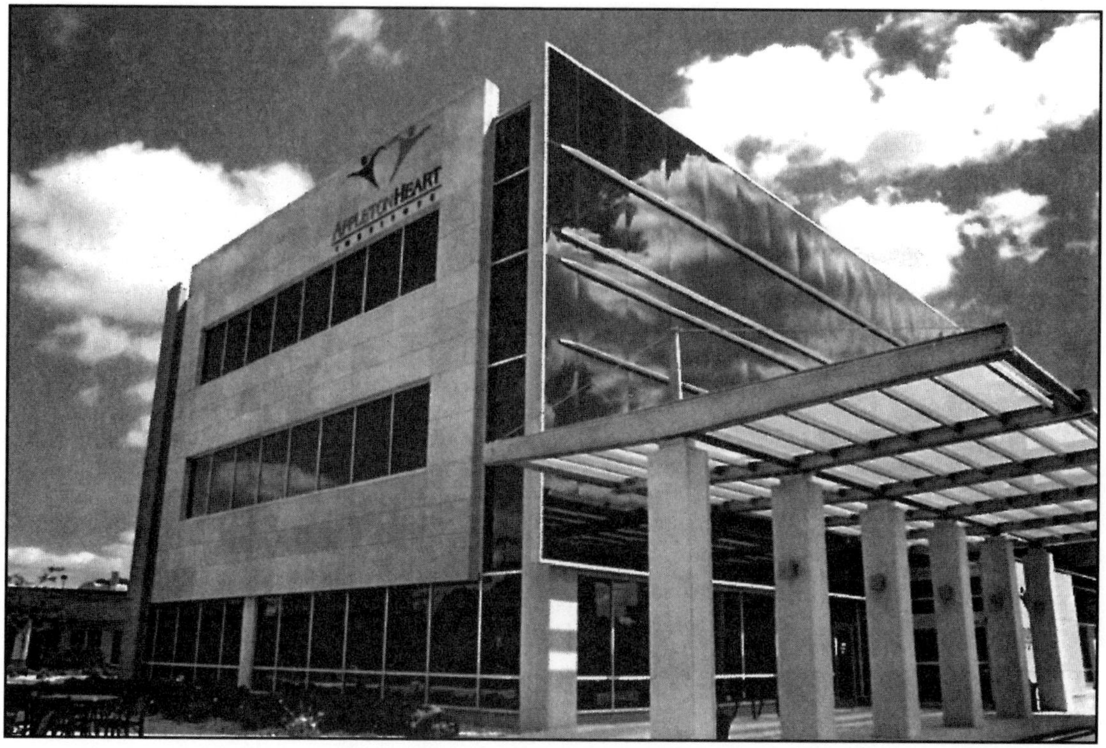

The new Appleton Heart Institute building

Chapter Twelve

THE GLORY YEARS

(1980-1988)

Leaving Internal Medicine Associates S.C. after ten years of total dedication to that group and its mission felt surreal, but at the same time I was never left adrift. With the addition of Dr. Cole in 1980, Dr. Mielke and I started again, this time focusing on creating the best cardiology practice in the area. Because Dr. Cole had expertise in nuclear cardiology, visualizing cardiac function and coronary arterial perfusion of heart muscle with radioisotopes was now possible. Combining nuclear imaging with treadmill exercise stress testing increased the sensitivity and specificity of this diagnostic study.

For my part, the latest advancement of technology and methodology of treating coronary artery disease came to me via a German physician and master showman. Andreas Gruentzig, working in Zürich, Switzerland, in the late 1970s, developed special catheters for dilating coronary arteries and eliminating obstructions. The procedure became known as PTCA (percutaneous transluminal coronary angioplasty) or balloon angioplasty. Gruentzig presented his technique and results at the American Heart Association Scientific Meetings in 1979, generating a great deal of enthusiasm as well as the expected skepticism. He was soon recruited to Emory University in Atlanta, Georgia, where he proved himself as an excellent technician, teacher, and promoter of the procedure. He gave live demonstration courses for cardiologists from around the world at Emory in the ensuing years. I went there twice for training and enlightenment on the procedural techniques and found Dr. Gruentzig to be a charismatic teacher, and yes, a showman, who would not only talk with the patient during the procedure, but also accept

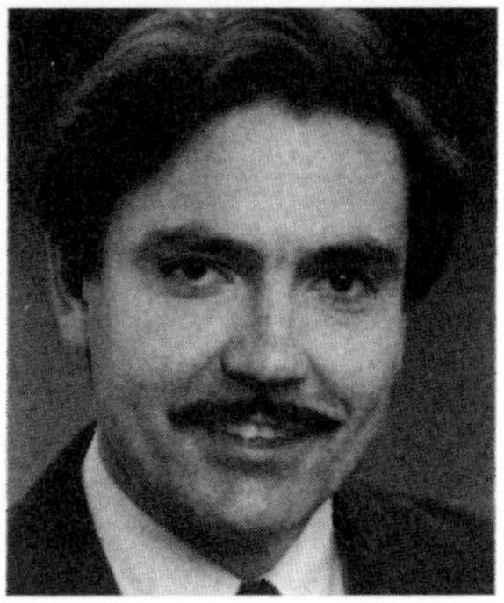

Dr. Gruentzig

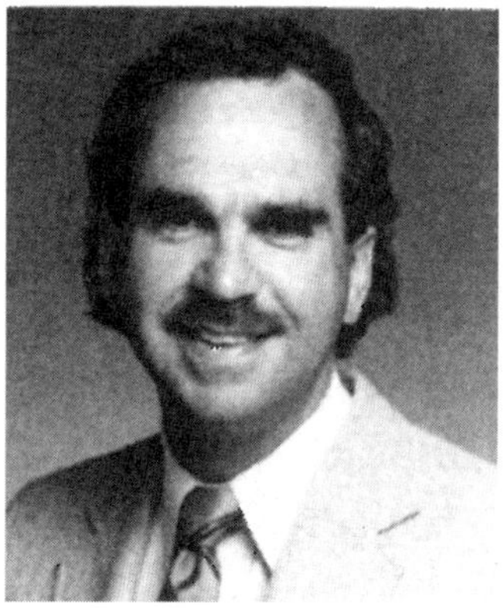

Dr. Hartzler

questions from the audience while he worked.

Cardiologist, Dr. Gerald Dorros, learned the angioplasty procedure from Dr. Gruentzig in Zürich and was actively performing these procedures in Milwaukee. I became aware of this and referred several patients to Dr. Dorros for balloon angioplasty. I observed his procedures on these patients. I also traveled to Kansas City to observe the work of Dr. Geoffrey Hartzler, a highly-skilled PTCA practitioner. With exposure to the skill of these talented interventional cardiologists, and by attending the live demonstration courses in Atlanta, I felt confident I was ready to perform the PTCA procedure in the catheterization laboratory at Appleton Medical Center. The technique was far from being as sophisticated as it is today. I only had a choice of two balloon catheters, each with a fixed, non-movable, short guide wire at the distal end, and the only size balloon available was about an inch long and 2.5-3.0 mm in diameter when inflated. The atmospheric pressure that could be exerted on these balloons was limited to eight to ten atmospheres and, if exceeded, the balloon would rupture and dissection (tearing of the inner lining of the coronary artery) occurred. This would inevitably lead to closure of the coronary artery with a thrombotic clot and therefore represented a surgical emergency for coronary bypass surgery. Significant advancements in balloon catheters and guiding catheters occurred over the next several years, including the development of balloons that could tolerate higher atmospheric pressure over prolonged inflations, and the so-called "over the wire" systems. This allowed flexible guide wires to be passed through a separate passageway of the catheter so that previously inaccessible blockages could be crossed. The balloon catheter could then be threaded over the wire and through the stenosis (narrowed artery segment caused by cholesterol plaque).

If anyone had told me early in my career that I would be threading wires and balloons down coronary arteries at minimal risk of complication, I would have told them they were crazy. But, for a period of about six years, I did just that. I carried out the first successful elective balloon angioplasty in the cardiovascular laboratory at Appleton Medical Center in January 1982. I enjoyed doing balloon angioplasty more than anything. The thrill of correctly positioning a balloon in a severely narrowed segment of a coronary artery and watching the balloon inflate into a sausage-link shape created by the narrowed segment of the artery, and then seeing that narrowing disappear as the increased pressure in the balloon crushed the plaque up against the wall of the artery, similar to a foot stepping on soft snow, was exhilarating. I used to call these successful procedures, "O-cases", because it gave me an orgasmic rush of excitement.

At about the same time that balloon angioplasty was in its infancy as an elective therapeutic endeavor and before PTCA was utilized as an emergency non-elective procedure for heart attacks, I learned about a new procedure called intra-coronary streptokinase infusion which was an emergency therapy for dissolving blood clots in the coronary arteries. The thrombolytic (clot dissolving) drug, streptokinase, could reestablish blood flow through the coronary artery, limiting the size of the myocardial infarction (heart attack) and increasing the patient's chance of survival. I recall being at the annual convention of the American Heart Association (AHA) and listening to Dr. Peter Rentrop, who pioneered the procedure, describe his technique, but he was being very cautious about promoting its extensive use. Dr. Gensini, a respected older invasive cardiologist stepped to the floor microphone to comment and exclaimed, "Peeta, Peeta, you are your own worst enemy!"

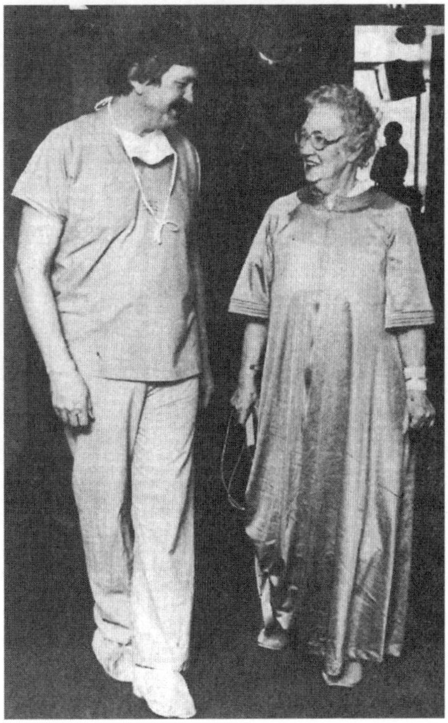

Me and my first successful angioplasty patient

Initially, I delivered the streptokinase directly into the coronary artery by placing a small catheter close to the clot through a guiding catheter and then slowly dripping the solution of streptokinase from an IV bag. This was very tedious and successful in only about 50 percent of cases. Sometimes the clot would dissolve rapidly and at other times I would just stand by for one to two hours and watch as the solution dripped in. When the clot dissolved and blood flow was restored, the patient would often go into ventricular tachycardia or ventricular fibrillation (totally erratic cardiac rhythms)

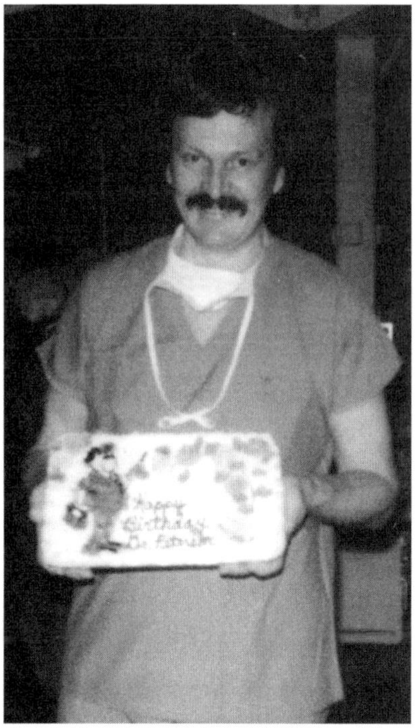

that were life-threatening and required electric shock defibrillation. I described these cases as hours of boredom interrupted by moments of sheer terror. Because these encounters took so long, often occurred at night, and involved acutely-ill patients, they were some of my most stressful cases.

It became apparent that infusing newer genetically engineered thrombolytic drugs intravenously through a peripheral vein could achieve similar results to that achieved by direct administration of streptokinase into the coronary artery. Therefore, this procedure could be carried out in emergency rooms or intensive care units rather than in the catheterization laboratory. Even with these advancements, the acute reestablishment of coronary flow and the overall successful patency rate was probably still about 60 percent.

On one occasion, I was treating a patient in the catheterization laboratory with intra-coronary streptokinase and elected to utilize a balloon angioplasty catheter to deliver the drug into the coronary artery. These catheters were very expensive, but I felt they were safer than utilizing a cheaper small caliber catheter because the small catheter was like a needle and could easily perforate the coronary artery. Suddenly, during the streptokinase infusion, the balloon catheter migrated right through the clot. I was stunned! If I tried to remove the catheter, I might pull the clot back and occlude the entire network of coronary arteries I was trying to protect. After assessing my options, I finally decided the best thing to do was inflate the balloon and crush the plaque and clot against the wall of the vessel. In essence, I ditched the Streptokinase procedure and proceeded with an acute angioplasty procedure. The balloon was then deflated safely and removed back into the guiding catheter. Further filming showed that the artery was now patent and oxygen-rich blood was flowing freely to the heart muscle. The clot was gone, and the patient was stable and pain free. Evaluation of his ventricular function, however, showed an akinetic (non-moving) anterior wall of the heart suggesting that the streptokinase infusion and balloon angioplasty were not

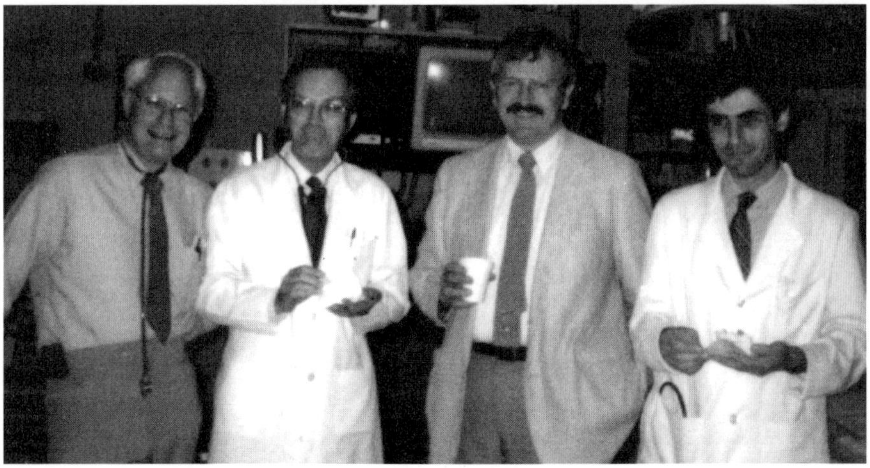

Left to Right: Doctors Mielke, Cole, Peterson, and Wilson

effective in salvaging his myocardium (heart muscle). The lack of muscle salvage in this case, and the concern about the safety of performing angioplasty in the setting of an acute myocardial infarction—which at this time had not been presented in the medical literature—prevented me from carrying out further similar procedures. PTCA in acute myocardial infarction would become commonplace and the well-established standard of care in years to come, but at this time it was just another fragile, scary footstep to the future.

I am very pleased I was able to treat many more patients, both acutely during myocardial infarction and electively for obstructive coronary disease, with angioplasty throughout the years that followed. For many of them the procedure was definitively successful and long lasting in relieving their angina and myocardial ischemia, and for others, it delayed by months and years their need for coronary artery bypass grafting (CABG).

In this "golden age of cardiology", the pharmaceutical industry developed new drugs that resulted in successful treatment of hypertension, angina, cardiac arrhythmias, congestive heart failure, stroke, peripheral vascular disease, and many other entities that were previously inadequately treated. Looking back, the 1970s and 1980s were medically mind-boggling.

By 1988 I was looking forward to seeing what other procedures and challenges were on the horizon, but life had other plans for me, and I suddenly found myself as a consumer rather than a provider of cardiac care.

Chapter Thirteen

THE OTHER SIDE OF THE STETHOSCOPE: ROLES REVERSE

(1988)

Denial, the bane of every cardiologist's practice, is predominantly but not exclusively, a male characteristic. After many years of practice, I realized denial could be included on a routine checklist of symptoms, right alongside headaches and heartburn. I have scolded countless patients to change their diets, behavior, or lifestyle, but rarely to great effect. Of course, when a patient doesn't believe there is anything wrong with his habits of daily living, it's difficult to administer preventive care. But, when they suffer an acute event such as a heart attack, they come up on the learning curve very quickly. If I've heard it once, I've heard it hundreds of times: "I didn't think it was anything, Doc; I just thought I had the flu," (or just as frequently—arthritis, rheumatism, a virus, or muscle spasms from exercise or overwork). Fortunately, these were the survivors of their acute coronary syndrome, who sheepishly related their stories, usually at the insistence of a concerned or nagging spouse. Tragically, for others stuck in denial, their first pain had been their last.

Denial is so ubiquitous, in fact, perhaps the irony of the next statement shouldn't surprise anyone: I thought heart disease would never happen to me. To this day, I rationalize it, saying truthfully, my symptoms were atypical. It did not seem possible or logical that my general lassitude, fatigue, tiredness, gastric upset, and excess gas and belching, had anything to do with my heart. I was so wrong.

In the fall of 1987 while raking my yard right after eating a large evening meal and having dessert of a delicious marital argument, I stopped in order to catch my breath, which in the spirit of denial, I blamed on age, poor conditioning, and stress. After a few minutes I resumed working and didn't think anymore of it. That winter I continued to work long hours and experience my usual fitful sleep (diagnosed years later as severe sleep apnea), and I generally did not feel well. But, wasn't that what hard working professionals should expect? I figured I could deal with it, and treated my symptoms with an increased consumption of my favorite medicine, gin. This not only elevated my spirits and dulled the symptoms, but it also heightened my state of denial.

By the spring of 1988, the jig was up. I felt so awful day after day I knew that I must be truly ill. I didn't have any idea what was wrong but I was betting on cancer. I concluded I could no longer blame everything on work-related stress.

I made up my mind that I needed a good physical examination and especially a good gastroenterology evaluation. I made an appointment for mid-May with Dr. Michael Geall, a former associate at Internal Medicine Associates, saying that I probably needed an abdominal ultrasound (reflected sound waves—from and to—a transducer on the abdominal wall drawing a picture of internal organs) and upper G.I. endoscopy (direct stomach visualization with a scope). I then left for a medical conference in Milwaukee where my wife and I enjoyed a very relaxing few days away from work. With the help of the requisite cocktail parties I even started to believe that I might not be sick after all. (It still amazes me how quickly denial can trump everything when given the chance.) Upon return, however, it only took me a couple of days to feel just as bad as I had before I left. Now, I was really scared. I called Mike's office and asked his assistant, Kathy, to move up my appointment and arrangements were made for me to be seen the following day. Mike performed a most thorough consultation and physical examination. My fate was in his hands. I knew he was as knowledgeable as any practitioner I had ever been associated with, as well as being an expert endoscopist. Mike proclaimed in his succinct style and British accent that he did not think my problem was G.I. related, but that we should proceed with the studies I had anticipated. These came back negative for cancer, ulcers, esophagitis, gastritis, duodenitis, pancreatitis, pancreatic cancer, or biliary obstruction. With that, Mike said my problems were likely cardiac and further investigation in this regard was advisable. I was relieved I did not appear to have cancer but was devastated by the thought that my symptoms were related to my own specialty! It is often said in medicine that, " a doctor who treats himself has a fool for a patient," and I had to face the fact that I had indeed been foolish.

I scheduled myself for a treadmill stress test with my associate, Dr. Cole. I was quite proud of myself, as I was able to go 13 minutes on the Bruce treadmill exercise protocol (taking me up to 5 mph at a 16 percent grade) without provoking chest pain. Still, the electrocardiogram revealed some mild suggestive abnormalities related to the inferior wall of the heart and Dr. Cole recommended that I have a nuclear imaging treadmill stress test. Again, I was able to accomplish 13 minutes without chest pain, but produced similar EKG findings. The nuclear thallium isotope scan of the heart was considered mildly abnormal, also on the inferior wall of the heart. Informed of the results, I knew that I was on a slippery slope and accelerating at a pace I still could not believe. Arrangements were made for me to have a cardiac catheterization carried out on Monday after completing these studies on Friday afternoon.

I was now faced with the unenviable task of telling my wife the results of the studies and that I would be undergoing an invasive procedure. The part I dreaded most was confessing the true nature of my symptoms, which I had dismissed for so long. She listened attentively and then proclaimed in her usual authoritarian manner that if the catheterization needed to be done, why would I wait until Monday? Get it done now! I was on weekend-call with Dr. Mielke and agreed to approach the subject with him the following morning. On Saturday morning, April 30, while making our morning rounds, I explained my wife's concerns, and therefore we agreed he would proceed with the catheterization and angiography study that same day. I completed my rounds, went to my office, cleared my desk of all the incomplete paperwork, filed my charges for work completed over the previous week, took a calcium channel blocker capsule and an aspirin, and with the casual air of a person familiar with the procedure, I confidently checked into the hospital. The whole situation was surreal and I kept telling myself there was at least a 50-50 chance the catheterization would not uncover any significant coronary disease.

My initial bravado quickly gave way to despair as I went through the routine steps of prepping for the diagnostic study. The initial laboratory blood-work obtained from a vein in my arm, the initiation of intravenous fluids into another vein, the placement of a hospital gown to replace my clothes, and a trip to the X-ray department in a wheelchair for a chest X-ray, as well as having my chest shaved, my arm and groin shaved, and further preoperative medications administered made me feel incredibly vulnerable. It wasn't that any of the procedures surprised me; I had seen patients go through the same prep hundreds of times.

But now that I was the one being poked and stripped, I was suddenly aware of my helplessness and this made each step acutely demeaning. Until that day, I never realized how I viewed myself as separate from those I treated—I was supposed to be the physician, not the patient. I couldn't help thinking about how many patients I had sent on a similar humiliating trip and had not had even a moment of remorse in doing so. This realization accentuated my despair.

I had requested our most experienced Cath. Lab nurse, Rosie Richter, be present for the procedure, as I trusted her implicitly and felt a whole lot more relaxed with her in the room along with our other very capable X-ray technicians and nurses. Following the procedure I was taken back to my room on 2-South at Appleton Medical Center. Shortly thereafter, Dr. Mielke entered the room to explain the results of the angiography. I was hoping for the best, of course, but at this point I no longer trusted my body to corroborate any wishful thinking. It was pointed out that the situation was serious: two of the three major blood vessels (LAD=Left Anterior Descending and RCA=Right Coronary Artery) that supplied my heart with blood were almost completely blocked with some additional blockages in diagonal branches off the LAD. I broke down and cried for the second time in my adult life. I remember feeling that it was unfair for me to have this problem at age 52. The shock of the moment soon gave way to anger. I was angry at myself for neglecting the control of my weight, diet, cholesterol, and stress. I just never felt I had time to pay attention to my health and now I was paying the price. Dr. Mielke left the room and I advised my wife that she should probably go home and call the children to let them know what was happening.

Within minutes, I experienced a persistent, unmistakable, attention-getting, oppressive, heavy-pressure chest pain. It was the first clear-cut anginal chest pain that I had ever had. I recognized it immediately. I rang for the nurse, who responded promptly, and I told her to give me a sublingual nitroglycerin tablet because I was having chest pain. I also requested that she call Dr. Mielke. Kathy, the red-haired nurse, was about as scared as I was, and was trembling so badly she could hardly get the nitroglycerin under my tongue. Fortunately, my chest pain subsided within minutes of taking the medication. I was placed on oxygen and given a beta-blocker medication and things seemed to settle down. Just when I thought the situation had stabilized and was confident it was going to remain stable, a second episode of angina occurred, which again was relieved after sublingual nitroglycerin. At this point I was moved to the intensive care unit for closer observation and was started on an IV (intravenous) nitroglycerin drip. My wife was notified and in the midst of all of this excitement returned to the hospital and remained at my bedside throughout the afternoon. In spite of all the ministrations, the anginal chest pains kept recurring, leading to a high-level conference between Dr.Mielke, Dr. David Warner, cardiac surgeon, and other members of our cardiology group, but I already knew what was in store for me. I could not see any way to resolve this situation safely without surgical coronary bypass. But, it was decided I should undergo a repeat cardiac catheterization to try and determine what was causing the instability of my clinical status. The procedure revealed an unstable ulcerated plaque in the proximal right coronary artery with some clot attached, and it appeared that the left ventricle of my heart was showing hypokinesis (decreased contraction) of the inferior wall, which would be compatible with abnormalities in the right coronary artery. It was determined I could no longer be treated medically and that there was no place for coronary angioplasty of this unstable lesion. Surgery was my only option.

Arrangements were quickly under way in the operating room to carry out emergency coronary bypass surgery. I had great confidence in Dr. David Warner and considered him to be among the best cardiac surgeons anywhere in the Midwest. I requested Dr. Chris Weinlander to be my anesthesiologist, even though he was not on-call, and he graciously complied. All of my children except my youngest, Erik, were living quite far away but were made aware of the situation through multiple telephone conversations with my wife. My father and brother were notified along with my wife's brother and his family. The shock waves of my situation resonated throughout the hospital and I recognized a palpable quiet among the nurses and staff as they came face to face with the reality of my impending surgery and uncertain outcome. I realized and cherished how important it was to have a strong support group of family, friends,

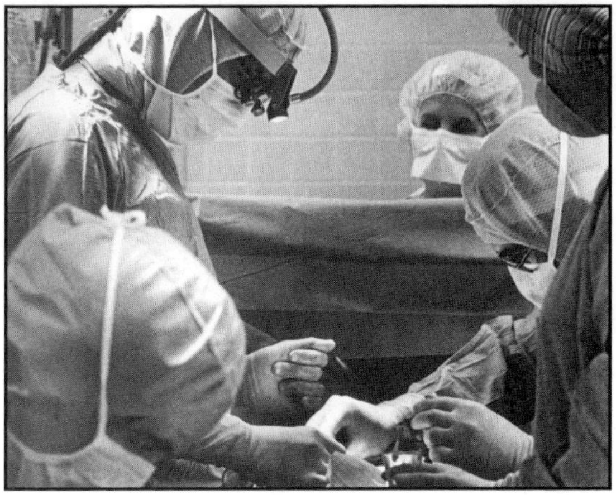

Dr. David Warner

and colleagues. I would not let the surgical team take me to the OR (operating room) until my son, Erik, could come to the hospital so I could tell him as a representative of all of my family how much I loved him. He covered the ten blocks to the hospital in no time flat on his skateboard.

The operating room crew and the surgeon were becoming impatient and worried that my situation would destabilize and then they would be faced with a much more serious and risky "crash" procedure. I felt sorry for them because I knew they were going to be in the operating room most of the night with me. After the initial prepping, washing, and shaving of practically my entire body in the OR, more IV fluid lines as well as an arterial line were placed. The anesthesiologist then administered intravenous medication that would markedly decrease my saliva and keep my airway dry and clean. He followed this with injection of propofol which is white in color and which I always refer to as the "milk of sleep". That is the last I remember until I awakened in the intensive care unit with the sun well up in the sky the next morning.

Apparently the surgery was anything but routine. After the administration of the propofol I was intubated successfully with an intra-tracheal tube and placed on the anesthesia-ventilator machine. During induction of anesthesia, however, I suffered a cardiac arrest with ventricular fibrillation. I was resuscitated with CPR and a defibrillation electric shock. After Dr. Warner entered my chest I was placed on the heart/lung pump oxygenator to support my circulation and red blood cell and tissue oxygenation. An attempt was made to bypass my right coronary artery with the right internal mammary artery (RIMA) which runs down the inside of the rib cage, but due to extensive calcification in the right coronary, the RIMA was found to be too short to reach the distal anastomosis site and it had to be ligated and abandoned. The left internal mammary artery (LIMA) was apparently quite huge and was easily anastomosed to the left anterior descending coronary artery. Saphenous veins from my left lower leg were harvested while the rest of the procedure was going on and these were then connected from my central aorta to the right coronary artery and to two diagonal branches of the LAD. After completion of the procedure and re-warming of my body temperature (cooled to Alaskan winter temperatures for preservation of the heart muscle during surgery), my heart was defibrillated to a normal rhythm and I was weaned from the heart/lung machine and stabilized prior to closing the chest.

I would remain under deep sedation with the endotracheal tube in place connected to a ventilator in the intensive care unit for several hours postoperatively. It is my understanding that after returning to the intensive care unit, I developed an arrhythmia that again required CPR and electrical defibrillation. Apparently the arrhythmias could not be controlled with the usual therapy of IV lidocaine but eventually stabilized with IV procainamide. There was concern that the etiology of the rhythm abnormalities was related to my heart still being ischemic (lacking oxygen) and that one of my grafts may have become obstructed with a clot, but further observation tipped the scales toward riding it out rather than going back to the OR.

I woke up very suddenly and became aware that it was morning and that I was still alive, but for a short time, probably not more than a minute or two, I realized that I was totally paralyzed and could not move a muscle, which frightened me more than anything I had experienced in the previous 24 hours. The paralysis subsided and I had full mobility of my body and my extremities but I was very sore. The discomfort was not only related to having had my chest opened and my ribs stretched to create exposure for the surgery, but also to enduring the chest compressions during my cardiac arrests. My wife came to my bedside as soon as I awakened and I realized she had spent the night at the hospital without sleep. I tried to reassure her with a thumbs-up to indicate that I was doing fine and she should go home and get some sleep. I could not imagine the stress she had been under through the night and during my cardiac arrest episodes. I was told later that Doctors Rattray and Suarez, our other cardiac surgeons, sat with Mary and comforted her through much of this ordeal, for which we are eternally grateful.

The ICU nurses administered some IV morphine to ease my discomfort and I quickly dropped off to sleep. The morphine, however, put me on a psychedelic trip that was like a nightmare and when I awakened it was sudden and confusing. I made up my mind that I did not want any more of that. Therefore, in spite of the tremendous pain and soreness in my chest and the fact that I had drainage tubes in my chest to drain out any accumulated postoperative blood or fluids, I decided the pain was preferable to the mental anguish. In the meantime, my endotracheal tube was removed which I counted as one of the biggest blessings of the early postoperative period. When in place it gives one the feeling of constantly being on the verge of choking. I refused any further morphine, but I asked Dr. Warner, who was also interested in holistic medicine, to bring me some of his music therapy tapes so I could try to relax. He graciously obliged before he returned home late that Sunday afternoon to try to relax and catch up on the sleep I had deprived him of for the previous 24 hours. The music tapes were extremely helpful in diverting my mind from my physical discomfort and I actually was able to doze periodically throughout the night, but I did find piano music, for some reason, was more disturbing than comforting. In addition, I noted I was significantly disturbed by the somewhat busy color design on the drapes surrounding my bed. These auditory and visual aberrations are unexplainable and were sensations I had never experienced previously. It also became quickly apparent in the postoperative period that I had experienced a new short-term memory loss, and I also find this unexplainable other than to blame it on the effects of surgery, anesthesia, and decreased oxygen to the brain during the cardiac arrests.

I was continuing to have nearly unbearable pain and both of my shoulders felt as if they were being torn from my body by some giant hand. The following day my attending doctors insisted I take pain medication in order to get some rest, and after some experimentation, I found I could tolerate a combination of Demerol and Valium very well. This not only took care of my pain, but gave me a very gentle sedation that was very comforting. I would lean very heavily on this combination for the next several days. On the third day following the surgery my chest tubes were removed, which was an uncomfortable, but short-lived experience that felt as if my heart and lungs were being pulled out along with the tubes. Later on, the wires that had been attached to my heart and brought out through the chest wall for any emergency pacing of my heart were also removed. This was not uncomfortable, but I felt as if my chest was being tickled from the inside. I eventually passed all my tests of in-hospital recovery that included having bowel movements, taking a shower, and being able to ambulate around the hallways three times in a row, and I was discharged home on the 11th postoperative day.

The tremendous outpouring of concern for me by the hospital staff, and by friends, relatives, and neighbors with flowers and cards was overwhelming. Some of the hospital maintenance staff even put up a sign on the roof of the first floor just outside my second floor window saying something to the effect of "Get well Dr. Peterson; Good luck". I remember vividly those who visited me. My wife drove me home from the hospital and although it was only a few blocks away it felt like a few miles. I slowly stepped out of the car in my driveway just as one of my former heart patients was walking by on the sidewalk. He apparently knew I had surgery and he stopped and commented, not encouragingly, that the reason I had this happen to me was because I was too damn fat. In my already depressed mood, I did not need to hear this. I was not only depressed, but I was angry, and I swore that I would never take care of that SOB again, as his simplification of my problem bordered on stupidity.

Phase two of my recovery began on an outpatient basis at Appleton Medical Center with rehabilitation sessions three times per week supplemented by exercise walking regimes at home the other four days of the week. With the weather improving, I transferred my cardiac rehabilitation sessions to Riverside Hospital at Waupaca and lived at my summer home on the Chain O' Lakes. As an example of how debilitated I was at this stage of my recovery, I remember being afraid to walk down to the lake or down the small hill leading into my driveway as I did not feel I had the energy, strength, or lung capacity to get back to the house. Gradually all of these things improved and I was able to walk at a brisk pace two to three miles, as well as work out on the treadmill and Air-Dyne bicycle at the rehab sessions at the hospital. I followed a low-cholesterol, low-saturated fat, weight reduction diet, lost about 25 pounds and gradually improved my strength. I was able to return to work in August 1988.

After extensive negotiations with my associates, and because of my desire to resume my cardiology practice, it was determined that I would no longer be expected to take night-call or weekend-call and would have to give up doing angioplasty procedures. I continued to do cardiac consultations, see patients in the office, do cardiac catheterization studies, and place permanent pacemakers until my retirement 22 years later. Because of the restrictions, I gradually reduced and eliminated emergency room coverage and intensive care unit coverage. As a result of this new arrangement my financial remuneration was reduced significantly such that I received 65 percent of what my partners earned. I also was required to cash out my accounts receivable. I insisted on maintaining my share of ownership of the corporation, and therefore my voting rights. Although giving up angioplasty was difficult, as I sincerely loved performing these procedures, my stress level was lowered. Most important, in spite of the significant financial and practice restrictions placed on me, my work schedule was reduced—from 60-100 hours to about 40 hours per week—which allowed me to continue to practice my profession comfortably, to the satisfaction of my patients at the Appleton Heart Institute, Appleton Medical Center, Theda Clark Hospital, and Riverside Hospital.

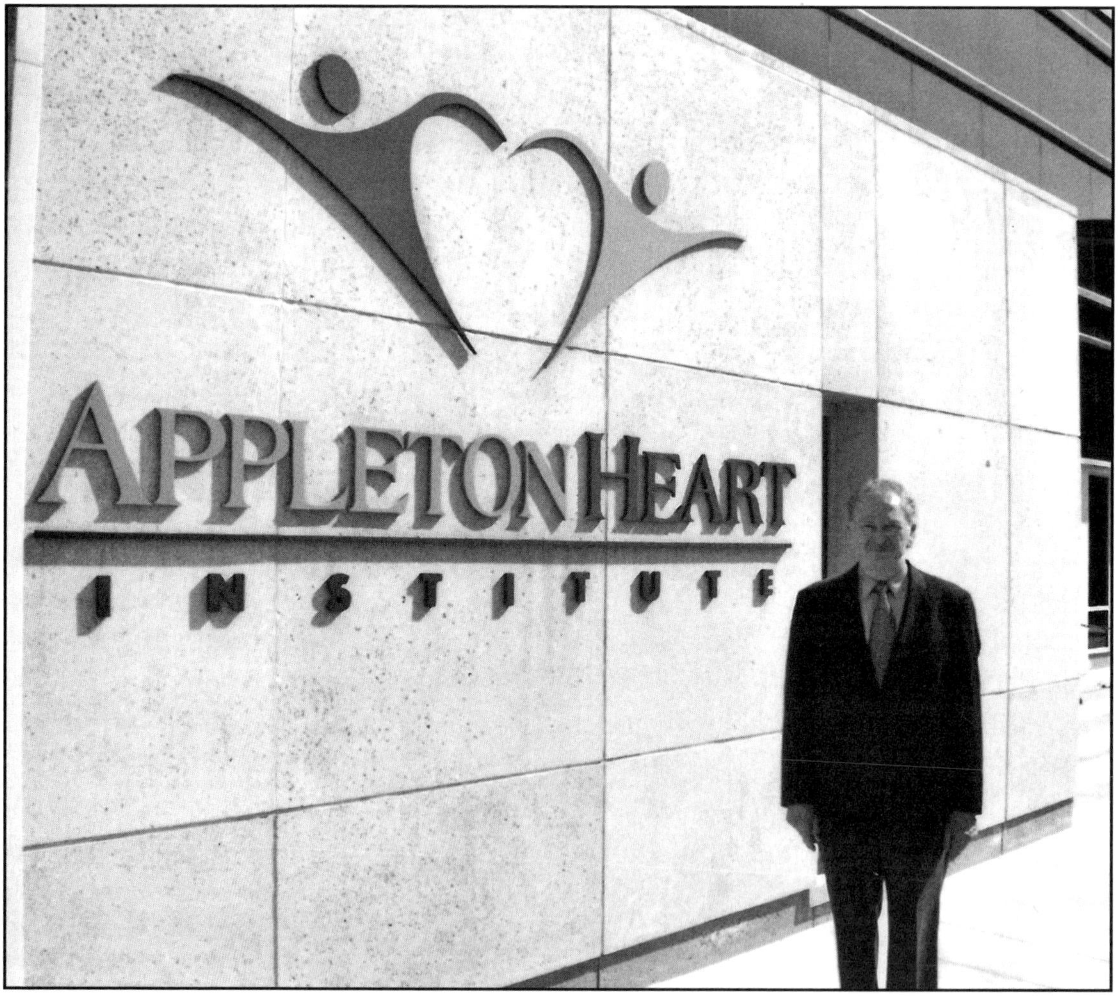

Me, on my retirement day, in front of the Institute I helped establish

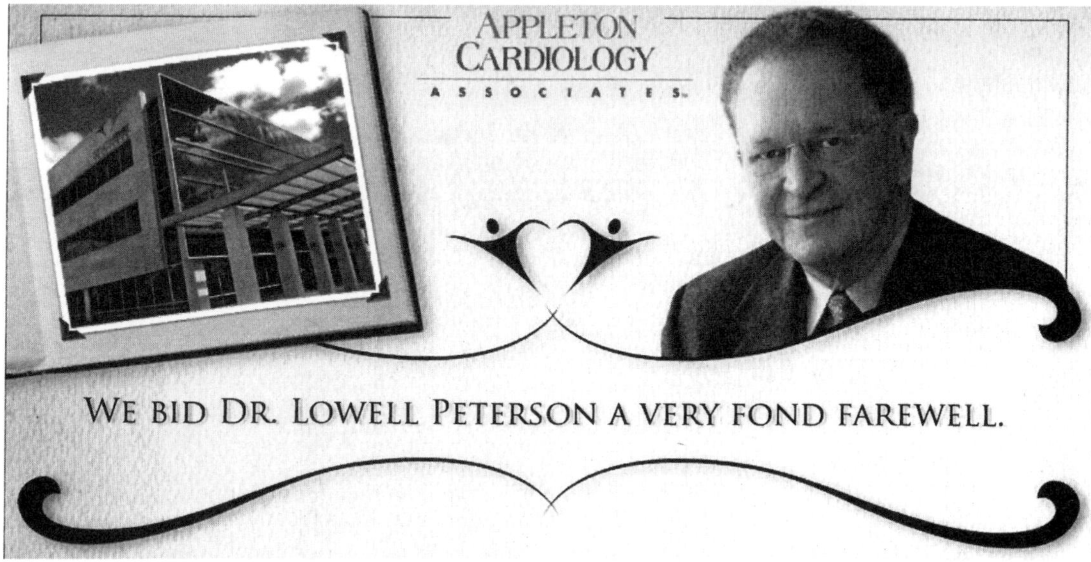

After having cared for patients for more than 38 years, Dr. Peterson will soon be putting his considerable energies into his retirement. While he'll no longer be an active part of our team, his remarkable contributions will continue to enhance this community.

Dr. Peterson was a pioneer in building the extensive range of cardiovascular services known today as the Appleton Heart Institute. Led by his vision, the Appleton Heart Institute has grown to become northeast Wisconsin's largest cardiovascular program, with offices in 11 communities beyond the flagship facility on the campus of Appleton Medical Center. Among Dr. Peterson's many accomplishments are establishing the area's first cardiac catheterization laboratory, developing a pacemaker implant program and spearheading the commitment to bring heart services to rural communities. Somehow he also found time to author three books; his writing continues to inspire us.

Dr. Peterson - or as your patients affectionately call you "Dr. Lowell" - you have the unwavering gratitude of both your colleagues and the community. It has been a great honor to have served with you. We offer our best wishes for a fulfilling retirement.

—Published by the Appleton Cardiology Associates

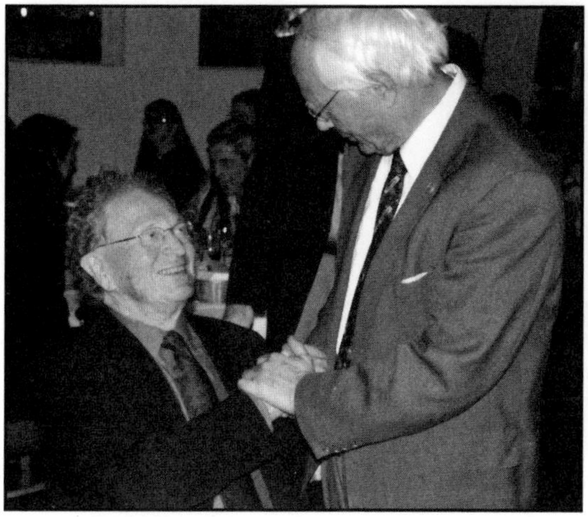

Dr. Mielke and me at my retirement party

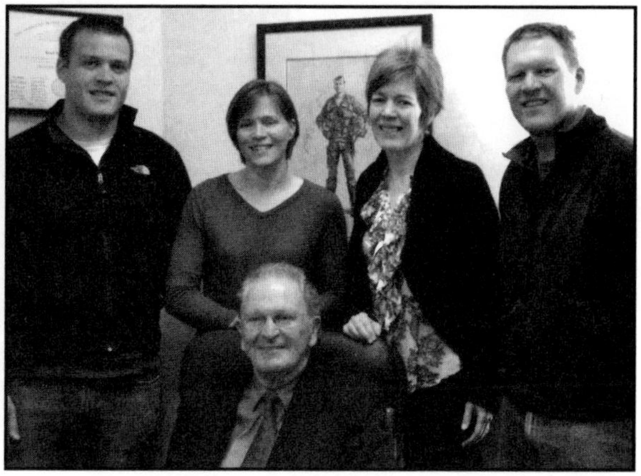

My last day in my A. H. I. office surrounded by my children; Erik, Kitty, Linda, and Jim

Chapter Fourteen

THE CULMINATION OF A LABOR OF LOVE

In 2008 I made a decision that the time had come to consider retirement from my practice of cardiology and from medicine in general. I was 72 years old, 20 years out from coronary bypass cardiac surgery, and I had accomplished most of my goals. It was time to pass the torch to the younger generation. One of my major career objectives was to establish, enhance, and maintain a viable cardiac consultation practice at Waupaca's Riverside Medical Center. After more than 35 years of diligently serving that community I now felt confident that when I stepped aside, the service would continue to thrive. Top-notch cardiologists, Dr. Michael Gitter, Dr. Brian Guttormsen, and Dr. Pat Mannebach would take over as cardiac consultants in this rural satellite hospital. (Did it really take three cardiologists and their physician assistants to replace me?) Not only would they replace me, they would enhance the service with their expertise. Saying goodbye to the medical and paramedical staff of Riverside Medical Center, Appleton Medical Center, and the Appleton Heart Institute, as well as saying goodbye to my faithful, pleasant, and loyal patients was very difficult. They were friends and family to me.

I feel that our group of cardiologists will continue to prosper based on the quality and quantity of services they provide. At the time of my retirement in February 2009, Appleton Cardiology Associates had five fully trained coronary artery PTCA providers who are also skilled in coronary and carotid artery stenting, peripheral arterial angioplasty, catheter closure of atrial septal defects and patent foramen ovales, as well as performing other diagnostic and therapeutic catheter procedures. The group also has two trained electrophysiologists capable of carrying out diagnostic arrhythmia studies as well as placing pacemakers, biventricular pacemakers, implantable cardiac defibrillators and performing ablations of rhythm abnormalities i.e. atrial flutter, atrial fibrillation, Wolf-Parkinson-White syndrome, and other congenital, concealed, electrical conduction pathway abnormalities. Multiple members of the group are involved in echocardiography, nuclear cardiology, and CT scanning of the heart and great vessels. Aside from the procedures, the clinical practice of cardiology at the Appleton Heart Institute, Appleton Medical Center, Theda Clark Hospital, and at all of the satellite hospitals served within a radius of 60 miles, continues to have the well-being of the patients at heart (no pun intended).

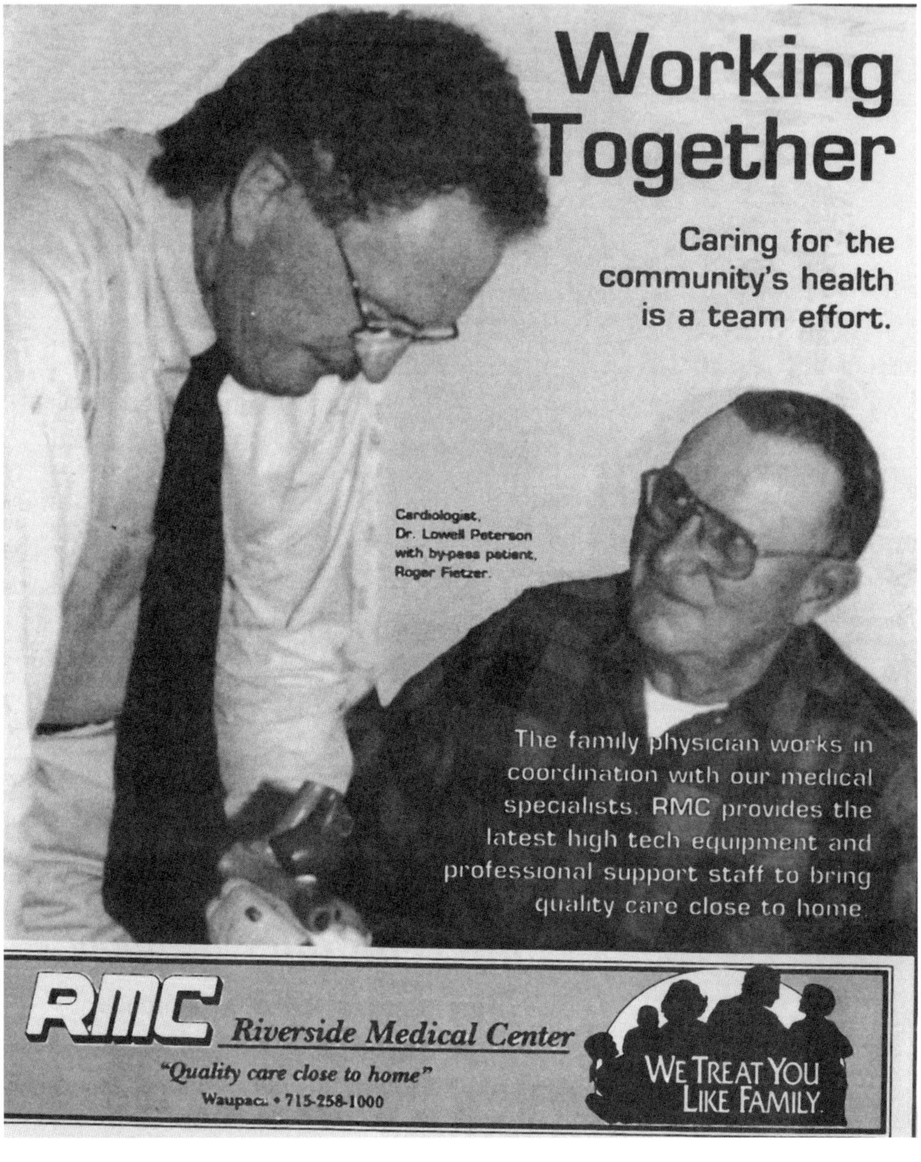

To be a part of the medical profession for almost 50 years has blessed me beyond anything words can describe. I feel privileged to record with words, my trip through my incredible, improbable journey. I am honored to have shared this journey with my family, my professional and paraprofessional medical colleagues, and my patients.

WAUPACA COUNTY POST JULY 28, 1994 PAGE 26

Health

Cardiac catheterization in great demand at Riverside

By PAUL JENSON

With heart disease the leading cause of death in Waupaca County, it is fitting that Riverside Medical Center has a comprehensive diagnostic cardiac care program to help area residents.

The convenience of having these high-tech, quality healthcare services close to home saves area residents the time and expense of traveling to an unfamiliar large hospital, plus the unfamiliarity of dealing with the city traffic.

Dr. Lowell Peterson, a cardiologist and associate of the Appleton Heart Institute, has been serving the Waupaca area through Riverside for the past 20 years. During this time he has seen the need for his consultation services grow dramatically. Responding to the need, he recommended the development of a comprehensive cardiac program.

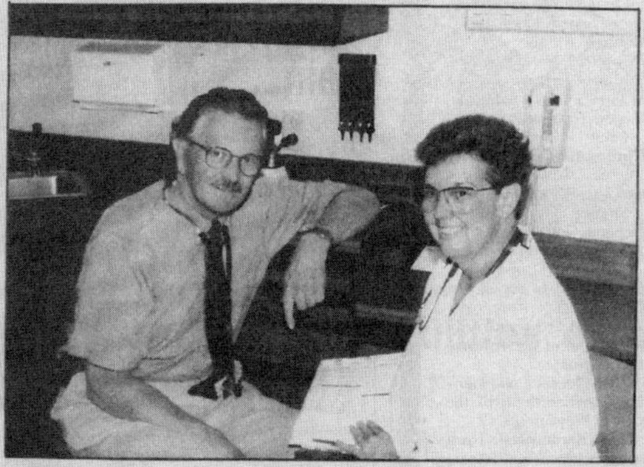

BUSY TIMES – Dr. Lowell Peterson and assistant Jean Lehndorf, a registered nurse, provide cardiology services at RMC, trying to combat the number one killer in Waupaca County. Peterson saw more than 700 patients in 1993. (Photo by Paul Jenson)

The cooperative effort by the RMC administration, Board of Directors and medical staff has resulted in a cardiac care program at Riverside that offers a vast number of services.

Cardiac catheterization is one of the high technology services available through this program. It is a common, nonsurgical method to help a patient's doctor diagnose a heart problem. To perform the procedure, a cardiologist inserts a long, flexible tube called a catheter into a blood vessel and guides it toward the heart. Once the catheter is in place, X-rays can help determine whether or not blockages are present in the coronary arteries. These and other tests are done to help doctors evaluate how well the heart is functioning. Cardiac catheterization is a unique service to the entire Central Wisconsin area.

The Appleton Heart Institute's Mobile Cardiac Catheterization Lab is a complete lab housed within a mobile unit. It contains the same equipment as located at Appleton Medical Center; the only difference is the fact it's on wheels.

Having a mobile unit allows patients to receive the most advanced care close to home and enables the local hospital and primary care physician to remain actively involved in patient care. Medical technology costs money, and having a mobile unit also helps contain the cost of health care by allowing hospitals in the region to share the expense. In addition to Waupaca, the Cardiac Cath Lab visits hospitals in Antigo, Two Rivers, Shawano, Berlin and Chilton.

For additional information concerning the Cardiac Cath Lab, call the RMC Central Scheduling Office, 258-1110.

VIGNETTES OF MEMORABLE PATIENTS

I evaluated and treated thousands of patients during my career, most of whom presented with rather straightforward diagnostic problems and required well-established therapeutic regimes. The encounters were always challenging and never boring. The following cases, however, presented a unique challenge. They are unforgettable: haunting; etched in my memory; never leaving.

One evening in late 1971, I was called to Theda Clark Hospital by Dr. Bob Dedmon to see a 13-year-old-girl who was critically ill. She was in severe congestive heart failure. Her lungs were filling up with fluid; she had a very rapid heartbeat; her blood pressure was barely obtainable; and she was nearly comatose. She was gasping for air and I could barely feel her faint rapid pulse—almost too fast to count. Each breath I listened to with my stethoscope sounded like crinkling plastic wrap due to the fluid in the air-pockets (alveoli) of the lungs. A very loud, roaring, continuous murmur was audible over the heart—almost without using a stethoscope—and it was also heard over her entire chest, neck, and back. I knew her situation was life-threatening. I asked Dr. Mielke to join me and, upon further examination, we both agreed that something very catastrophic had happened to her aortic valve (the valve that protects the blood from flowing back into the heart once it has been pumped forward). The valve was severely insufficient, allowing blood pumped out of the heart to regurgitate back into the heart, creating the diastolic (during heart muscle relaxation) heart murmur. This put a massive strain on the left ventricle. In addition, a systolic murmur (during heart muscle contraction) likely represented a shunt across a ventricular septal defect—VSD— (a hole in the heart septum allowing blood from the left ventricle to cross to the right ventricle). I arranged for her immediate transfer to Appleton Memorial Hospital and alerted Dr. Hal Harding to prepare for emergency open-heart surgery. At surgery he found an overwhelming left-to-right shunt through a large VSD and leaflets of the aortic valve were prolapsing through the VSD allowing regurgitation of blood from the aorta back to the left ventricle, but also into the right ventricle through the VSD. This created a huge blood volume overload of the right ventricle and pulmonary circulation. Dr. Harding closed the VSD with a patch and replaced the leaking aortic valve, a highly technical feat in someone this critically ill. Just getting her on the heart-lung oxygenator pump and off again were major undertakings. Postoperatively, the patient remained in very critical condition. It became apparent she had suffered a stroke, maybe as a result of ischemia (lack of oxygen) or an embolus (air bubble or clot) to the brain during surgery. She died on the second postoperative day. This experience just drained me. Thirteen-year-old children are just not supposed to suffer such catastrophic illnesses and go from being well and vibrant with their whole life in front of them to becoming a casualty without a future in just 48 hours. I did what I could for her, but unfortunately it was not enough.

♥

In the late 1970s, I referred an elderly lady for coronary bypass surgery and replacement of her mitral valve. I had known her and her husband personally for many years as neighbors, but in later years I cherished them as my patients. The surgery seemed to go very well without complication, but the patient did not wake up after surgery and I suspected she had suffered a stroke. The neurology service doctors examined her thoroughly and found no evidence of brain function and held out little hope for her survival. There was total absence of reflexes, absence of response to painful stimuli, and an abnormal electroencephalogram (EEG)—brain wave—examination. A repeat examination 24 hours later showed no improvement and the neurology doctor declared her brain dead and suggested that, with the family's permission, the pulmonary ventilator (respirator) and the drugs that were supporting her blood pressure could be discontinued. Because of my emotional attachment to the patient nurtured by years of caring for her medically and knowing her family, I was not ready to give up. I insisted on examining the patient myself. During the examination I was surprised to find a single corneal blink reflex upon light touch to the left eye. I checked it repeatedly to be sure I was not imagining something that I wanted to be present. But, I wasn't imagining it: she definitely winked. I therefore vetoed the pronouncement of death and after discussion with the cardiac surgeons, neurologists, and the family, we decided to wait at least another 24 hours. For some miraculous reason more reflexes began to become active and more and more sensory and motor activity was elicited. The patient eventually awakened and made a complete recovery. I continued to provide her medical care until her death from old age. I am still baffled by her spontaneous recovery. Some would say it was a miracle; others, that "It just wasn't her time to go;" and scientifically one might speculate on a very slow metabolic recovery of body function from the stress of surgery, anesthesia, etc. As for me, I choose to leave it with the unknown and unexplainable, an event that requires faith and acceptance.

♥

I have seen several patients with Idiopathic Hypertrophic Subaortic Stenosis: (IHSS) or what is now called Hypertrophic Obstructive Cardiomyopathy (HOCUM). This is a congenital and often familial abnormality of muscle overgrowth in the left ventricle of the heart just below the aortic valve which can lead to partial obstruction of blood flow from the left ventricle into the aorta as the heart squeezes during systole. With increased heart rate (which accentuates the obstruction) associated with stress or activity, sudden death, especially in young athletes may occur. For several years I followed two young women as patients with this condition. Their situation seemed to be stable on medical therapy (to prevent tachycardia and decrease forcefulness of cardiac contraction). They were doing well and there did not appear to be any urgent reason to consider surgical removal of the overgrown muscular obstruction. However, I was unprepared for the shocking news when I received back-to-back phone calls—on the same day—that both of them had died suddenly. The one lady lived in a rural area and her husband, returning to the farmhouse from his morning chores in the barn, found her dead in bed. The second lady lived near Appleton and was a nursing instructor at the Fox Valley Technical Institute. She was simply walking down the hallway when she had sudden cardiac arrest and sudden death. Because there were students and faculty of an EMT and paramedic training program in the building, she was promptly attended to with CPR, but to no avail and she was pronounced dead. My emotions and reaction to these fatalities stressed my confidence as a cardiologist to the limits. I was consoled only by my knowledge that I was dealing with a potentially fatal disease from the get-go and the patients understood that as well.

♥

A patient presented to me at Riverside Hospital complaining of severe pain in his calves associated with walking. I thought he probably had blockages in his leg arteries because that is the most common cause of claudication (effort induced calf pain due to decreased arterial blood flow to the muscles). I fully expected to find he had diminished or absent pulses in his legs and feet, but when I examined him carefully, I found he had good pulses in his lower extremities. The history and the physical examination did not jibe. I was confused. But, the history was so strong for claudication that I saw no other choice except to evaluate him further with an arteriogram. I ordered the usual preoperative laboratory evaluation prior to proceeding with the arterial studies. The blood work revealed that his hemoglobin was less than 5 gms (normal 12-15 gms). This was the lowest hemoglobin I ever saw on someone not actively bleeding, except for a similar result in a Hindu woman I treated as an intern who was a vegetarian, not eating red meat, and at the same time losing blood chronically through monthly menstruation. The oxygen-carrying capacity within the hemoglobin of the reduced number of red blood cells became so severely limited that, with any activity, the muscles of the calves were starved for oxygen, leading to pain. So now, instead of looking for arterial blockages, I had to figure out why he was so anemic. I ordered further tests that determined he had pernicious anemia due to vitamin B-12 deficiency. My patient had been consuming enough B-12 in his diet, but he wasn't absorbing it in his distal small bowel because there was an absence of intrinsic factor produced by the parietal cells of the stomach. Atrophy of the parietal cells in the stomach leads to an absence of intrinsic factor and hydrochloric acid (HCl). If this situation is allowed to go on without replacement of the vitamin B-12, not only anemia occurs but neurologic involvement of the spinal cord may also occur. Even if the vitamin B-12 levels are replaced, the achlorhydria (absence of HCL) in the stomach may be a precursor to adenocarcinoma (stomach cancer). With this knowledge, I replaced the patient's vitamin B-12 levels after initial blood transfusions. Clinically he did very well. I followed him very closely every six months with X-rays and endoscopy looking for any evidence of stomach cancer. None was found until a couple of years later when a definite gastric cancer was present. The patient succumbed to his cancer. Sometimes, no matter how thorough the evaluation, treatment, and follow-up, the end result may not be optimal. I had to learn to accept this and live with it.

❤

A young boy of 10 to 12 years of age presented with chronic kidney disease probably from a significant previous episode of infectious inflammation of the kidneys (glomerulonephritis). He not only had chronic kidney disease and renal insufficiency (failure of the kidney's ability to clear wastes) but he had also developed renal osteodystrophy (a loss of bone formation) which leads to growth retardation and bowing of the long bones of the legs (Rickets). There is a loss of function of osteoblasts (the bone forming cells), decreased calcium absorption in the gut, and metabolic acidosis (lower pH than normal) that enhances bone reabsorption. All of this leads to decreased Vitamin D and onset of secondary hyperparathyroidism (overproduction of hormone from the parathyroid gland that further accelerates bone resorption). The hyperparathyroidism and the Vitamin D deficiency lead to the medical condition, Rickets. I treated this boy vigorously as an outpatient with 25-OH cholecalciferol Vitamin D and with phosphate binders and followed him very carefully in the office. To my amazement his bowed legs straightened, he actually gained some height, but he had no improvement in his kidney function. Because he had numerous siblings that I thought might provide a donor for renal transplant, I had him evaluated at the renal transplant service at Milwaukee County General Hospital. It was their feeling that the patient could continue to be treated medically.

This proved to be unfortunate because within the next year the patient developed an acute influenza episode which was complicated by Reye's Syndrome. This condition occurs in children and is often associated with aspirin use for the treatment of the flu symptoms. It is an acute encephalitis and encephalopathy (inflammation of the brain). My patient became totally psychotic with the acute episode, screaming profanities constantly, with his whole body writhing about the bed such that he required restraints and marked sedation. This condition again resulted in a transfer to Milwaukee County General Hospital for a plasmapheresis (blood cleansing) and exchange transfusions of almost his total blood volume. Although he recovered from the Reye's Syndrome, he was no longer a candidate for renal transplantation, because with the multiple transfusions, he now had acquired enormous numbers of foreign antibodies in his bloodstream not there before the illness and this would almost certainly lead to rejection of any transplanted organ. I think he discontinued his medications and he was lost to follow-up. I saw him at a local baseball game later that year and noticed his legs were again severely bowed. I presume he did not survive for any extended period of time.

❤

A patient came to my office who is impossible to forget. As he sat next to my desk, he was between me and a full-length mirror on the door. He conversed with me while watching himself in the mirror, making twitchy shadow boxing moves almost constantly. He told me he had been an amateur boxer in his younger days and I quickly concluded that he was "punch-drunk". He was very content living in his own little world. I cared for him medically for many years and when he finally came for coronary bypass surgery, he accepted it reluctantly based on the trust he had in me, aided by the urging of his delightful wife. During his recovery from his surgery, he laid in his bed with the lights off, because he was afraid to touch the switches for fear of electrocution. In spite of his erratic behavior, I got along with him very well, and enjoyed his visits and jovial conversation—but it made me introspective as to my own sanity.

❤

I was asked to see a patient at St. Elizabeth's Hospital because of a profoundly slow heart rate (bradycardia) with heart rates often as low as 20 beats per minute with long pauses that seemed to be asymptomatic. Examination revealed a significant heart murmur compatible with insufficiency (leakage) of the mitral valve. The patient was not at all concerned about his heart because he said that everybody in his family had heart problems and several had died at a young age. It became apparent his family suffered from a familial genetically transmitted cardiomyopathy (abnormal function of the heart) manifest by bradycardia (slow heart rate), significant mitral valve prolapse (floppy valve leaflets) leading to mitral insufficiency, as well as having physical features of a condition that weakens the walls of arteries. Over the next several years I placed permanent pacemakers in multiple members of this family for their bradycardia. My initial patient of this family later suffered a cardiac arrest, was resuscitated, and then had coronary bypass surgery and mitral valve replacement. The laissez-faire attitude toward the medical problems and the uncertain prognosis of these family members may actually have been a blessing.

♥

I was asked to see a man with a severe cardiomyopathy (heart muscle weakness) and intractable congestive heart failure not responding to medical therapy. He was moribund, totally bedridden, and functional class IV (comfortable only at complete bed rest). He exhibited cardiac cachexia (extensive muscle wasting and weight loss related to his chronic disease). I also observed cardiac Cheynes-Stokes respiration (periodic breathing), a sign of extremely low cardiac output and slow circulation time. After initial stabilization of the situation, I concluded he would only be helped by cardiac transplantation. I made arrangements to place him on a high priority list for transplant. Fortunately, a donor heart became available within a few weeks and the surgery was carried out successfully at the University of Wisconsin Hospital. The patient recovered and rehabilitated very nicely. He regained his weight and muscle strength, no longer appearing cachectic. He returned to operating his service station, but eventually sold it, remarried, and moved south to enjoy retirement with his new wife.

♥

A lady with high cholesterol, and a former smoker, developed severe diffuse vascular disease at a very young age, in her 20s. Over the ensuing years, she had numerous vascular operations to restore blood flow to her legs, her heart, and her brain, as well as catheter interventions with angioplasty of vessels. Obviously, a significant genetic factor was present in the propensity to develop such severe vascular disease, especially in a young female. Her positive attitude in spite of adversity was paramount in her survival and functioning. At my last encounter with her, she was relatively asymptomatic. She remarried and was enjoying going to dances at least twice a week. It is amazing to see these "vasculopath" survivors who have such severe atherosclerotic problems in so many vessels. I cared for other patients who only had one of four arterial blood vessels patent to their brain. I allowed them to have high blood pressure in order to provide a perfusion pressure to feed the entire brain through this single diseased artery. If the pressure got too low they would seizure and pass out. Fortunately, these patients are an anomaly to the usual atherosclerotic patients I encountered.

♥

A patient of mine was admitted to 4-North at Appleton Medical Center for flu and pneumonia. It was at a time when oral mercury thermometers were kept at every bedside in tiny glass vases filled with isopropyl alcohol. The nurses thought it was rather unusual that every morning when they went to take the vital signs of the patients, including taking their temperature, the alcohol vials were empty. They soon were able to deduce it was my patient who was walking the floors at night, going into all of the patient's rooms, and drinking the alcohol in the containers. I thought it was rather clever and hilarious, but the nurses and hospital administration were less inclined to deal with it in a jocular fashion.

♥

A patient whom I followed for many years because of severe aortic valvular stenosis (calcium hardened, immobile valve leaflets) also had markedly elevated total cholesterol of over 400 (normal-less than 200). But, his HDL-cholesterol (good cholesterol) was always greater than 100 and that is very high. He had several cardiac catheterization studies to evaluate his aortic valve for possible surgery and he did have a balloon catheter valvuloplasty (balloon dilatation of the valve) that was partially successful. He later had valve replacement. On each of the catheterizations, his coronary arteries were also evaluated by angiography and each time it was noted that his coronary arteries were totally normal without evidence of atherosclerosis. Therefore, I did not treat him with any Statins (cholesterol-lowering medications), because I felt that his high HDL was protecting him as well as any medication could. He lived into his mid-90s and died of old age with a heart and mechanical aortic valve that were working just fine until the end. He did however, in his later years, develop atherosclerotic disease of the blood vessels of his lower extremities which did cause claudication (calf pain). Therefore, he apparently was not totally protected from the ravages of high cholesterol by his high HDL.

♥

I admit to some carousing in the bars and dance halls of central Wisconsin during my college and early medical school years. During these escapades, my friends and I became acquainted with a group of girls, from a neighboring town, in one of our favorite hangouts, and after the bar would close at 1 a.m. or 2 a.m. we would often go to one of the girls' homes, go into the basement recreation room, eat snacks, play pool and ping-pong, and in general, just be noisy. On one of these occasions, the father of my girlfriend came down to the basement, rather angry, and told us all to go home because he had to work the next day and he was not getting any sleep. Approximately 20 years later when I was in practice I was asked to see this man as a patient in the hospital at Waupaca after he suffered a small heart attack. I recognized his name and silently hoped he had forgotten mine. I walked into his room and was about to introduce myself when he said, "I remember you, you are one of the S___s a' B_______'s that I threw out of my basement at three o'clock in the morning!" We both had a good laugh as I acknowledged my involvement. He lived many more years and I managed his cardiac problems with multiple medications which allowed him to continue to function through his retirement. Unfortunately, he developed a cancer that was incurable and was causing him a great deal of pain and suffering. Being a smart man, a professional man, he personally elected to discontinue all his cardiac medications and he soon died a cardiac death.

♥

The first permanent pacemaker I implanted at Appleton Memorial Hospital in 1970 was in an elderly gentleman with complete heart block and significant bradycardia. Thereafter, he lived several enjoyable retirement years in his home community and had more than one pacemaker generator change by me during that time. He eventually entered a nursing home and was very depressed by his failing health. He refused any further pacemaker generator changes. It was reported by the nursing staff at the nursing home that he would sit looking out the window as a hearse would pull away with someone who had expired during the previous night and he would say, "Don't go, wait for me." As comical as this may sound, we may all face a time in our life when the comfort of death may supersede our desire to live.

♥

In 1951, a British physician described a syndrome consisting of multiple-related psychiatric symptoms he named, "The Munchhausen Syndrome". This symptom complex was named for Baron von Munchhausen, a scalawag who lived in the 18th century and was known for relating fantastic and impossible adventures about himself. Persons who have the Munchhausen syndrome feign illness, or exaggerate symptoms to create a perception of illness for the purpose of drawing attention or sympathy to themselves. This often results in extensive medical investigations, treatment, and sympathy from medical personnel. Individuals with this syndrome are often very knowledgeable about the practice of medicine, describing their symptoms in detail. The simulation of disease is the central activity of the affected person's life. Munchhausen patients know they are exaggerating symptoms, whereas hypochondriacs believe they actually have a disease, and malingerers fake illness or symptoms for secondary gain such as to avoid work, but their condition is not pathologically psychiatric.

On a Sunday morning in the 1970s I was called to an emergency consultation on a patient in the intensive care unit who was felt to be having a myocardial infarction (heart attack). This middle-aged man described to me classical symptoms of angina pain that had accelerated in severity to a significant level such that he sought medical attention in the emergency room. He was promptly admitted, attended to appropriately with oxygen, nitroglycerin, monitoring, and placement of intravenous fluid lines for emergency medicine infusion if necessary. After completing my examination and reviewing his electrocardiogram (that was perfectly normal—as were his laboratory studies), I became suspicious that his illness was a ruse, possibly to receive narcotic medications. In addition, he just did not look very ill and even smiled as he presented his classical symptoms. I informed him I did not believe he was having a heart attack and that we would only be keeping him for observation until the following day. A telltale sign of the Munchhausen syndrome is often multiple scars on the abdomen from previous unnecessary operations, which he also exhibited. In spite of him switching some of his symptoms to abdominal pain rather than chest pain, I continued to refuse his requests for further intervention and insisted only on continued observation. He then became very angry and abusive, threatening to report me and the nurses to the authorities, and to sue us. I was not threatened by this and so informed him. He promptly took off his monitors and oxygen, had his IV lines removed, asked for his clothes, and promptly signed out AMA (against medical advice).

The hospital administration was advised of this case promptly, especially in view of the fact that he had threatened a lawsuit. They made inquiries of other hospitals in our area and throughout the state and found he had been in many hospitals in the recent weeks with similar symptoms. Munchhausen syndrome is often also referred to as the "hospital addiction syndrome", or the "hospital hopper syndrome". He certainly qualified.

I did not know where he went when he left the hospital but all hospitals within 50 miles were advised to be on the lookout for someone of his description and a believable symptom complex. The following day I was informed that a man fitting the description of my patient was killed by an automobile as he hitchhiked along Highway 41 toward Green Bay. It was reported that the man had actually stepped in front of the car as it slowed prior to coming to a stop to give him a ride. He had carried his need for illness or injury to gain attention and sympathy one step too far.

The intensive care unit at St. Elizabeth's Hospital in the early 1970s was a very crowded facility with five beds, a nursing station, and a bank of monitors. The rooms were small and gathering around a patient's bed in the heat of a crisis by physicians, nurses, and other paramedical personnel became a real challenge in the delivery of care. Because it was a Catholic hospital and the vast majority of the patients were Catholic, I would often ask the nurses to call the priest from his quarters to come and administer last rites. The priest was a small man with horn-rimmed glasses who always wore a plain black priest's robe. He would arrive promptly even in the middle of the night, stand outside the room, apply his religious sash about his neck, take out his prayer book, and begin to mumble his prayers as he entered the room where we were engaged in a battle for the patient's life. He would continue to mumble his prayers, never breaking stride as he circled the bed, gave the sign of the cross, and left the room. He removed his sash, put his prayer book back in his pocket, and disappeared. The entire Sacrament took less than one minute, but I am sure the patient (if they recovered), and the family of the patient were comforted by knowing the priest had ministered the last rites. They also were thankful we had been considerate enough in the heat of battle to ask for this religious blessing. The tremendous ability of the St. Elizabeth priest and the Catholic and Protestant chaplains at Appleton Medical Center to comfort the patients and their families should not be underestimated. This applies to the clergy of our extended area community as well. The calm ministry and compassion they provided made my job a whole lot easier.

THE APPLETON HEART INSTITUTE—
THE BIRTH OF A DREAM

The Appleton Heart Institute encompasses the labor of many people from the past, the day-to-day medical realities of the present, and the imaginative dreams of the future. The development of the Appleton heart program over the last 35 years of the 20th century coincides with the era best described as, "The Golden Age of Cardiology".

The visionary concept and subsequent development of the cardiovascular catheterization laboratory was accepted by the Appleton Memorial Hospital Board of Directors based on the faith the community had in its healthcare facilities and its providers. The first catheterization studies carried out in NE Wisconsin were performed by cardiologists, Dr. John Mielke and Dr. Lowell Peterson in August 1970. Thereafter, the natural evolution and growth of cardiac services led to the development of an open-heart surgery program. The first cardiac surgical coronary bypass operation was performed in August 1971. By 1989, 10,000

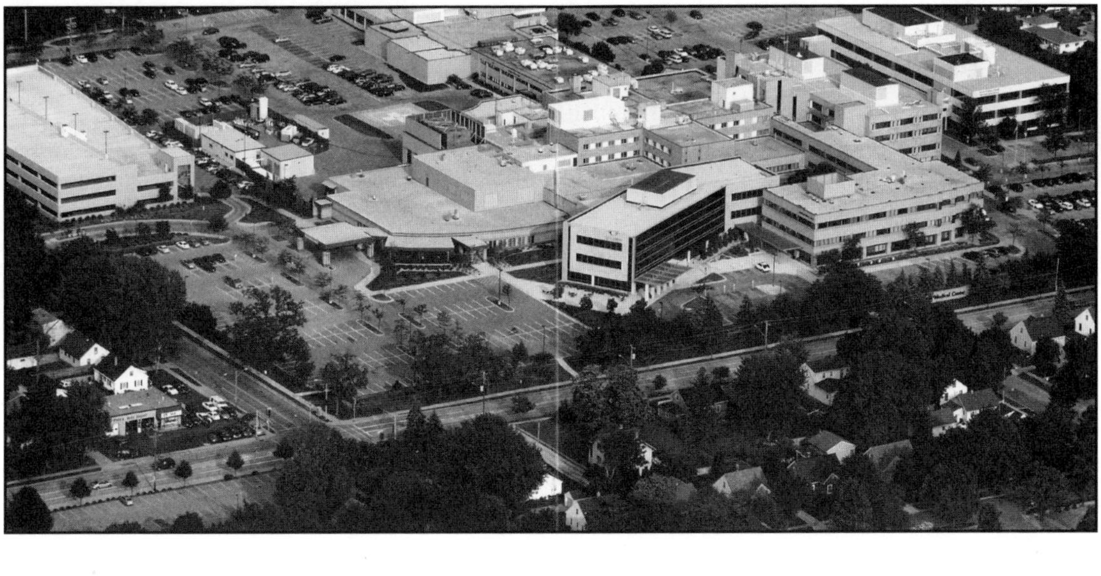

patients had been studied by cardiac catheterization. That number is currently approaching 50,000. At the present time there are four state-of-the-art catheterization laboratories functioning at Appleton Medical Center on a daily basis.

In 1982, Percutaneous Transluminal Coronary Angioplasty (PTCA) was successful for the first time at AMC, and the first stent procedure of a coronary artery was performed in July 1993. Stenting is currently the interventional procedure of choice for patients presenting with an acute myocardial infarction (heart attack), as well as being an adjunct to most angioplasty procedures.

The concept of a Heart Institute was born in 1982 after I visited the University of Minnesota and discovered their cardiology service had its own building, an entity easily identifiable by signage, that said, Minneapolis Heart Institute. The AMC governing board accepted my recommendation to follow a similar path and in a news release on November 1, 1983, Paul Groth, Chairman of the governing board, said, "The hospital has dedicated a significant portion of its resources and efforts over the past 15 years to its cardiovascular treatment program. The formation of the Appleton Heart Institute is a natural result of that continued dedication to high-quality cardiovascular care, and the hospital's commitment to innovatively and efficiently meet the consumer's needs for enhanced quality, convenience, and service."

Although motives were sincere, establishing a true identity of the Heart Institute, dedicated to formally combining and providing all cardiac services, was, for many years, not easily recognizable. With the opening of the Appleton Heart Institute (AHI) building in 2003, the dream was realized. The hard work and the faith in our efforts was now reality. The success of AHI and its physicians will continue to be judged by the public and by our peers in the future.

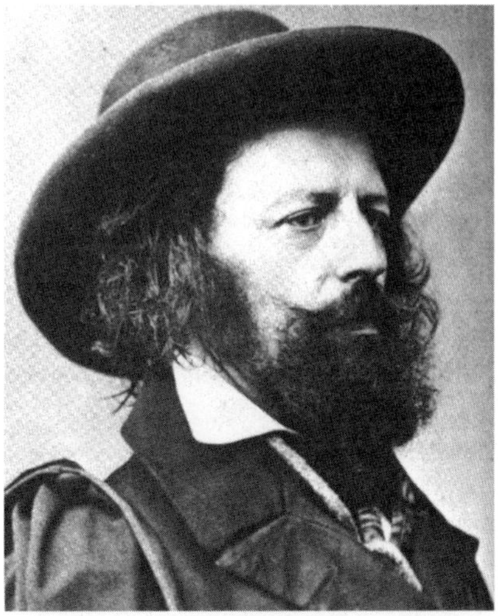

"Old-age hath yet his honor and his toil; death closes all:
But something ere the end, some work of noble note,
may yet be done, not on becoming men that strove with Gods.
The lights begin to twinkle from the rocks:
The long day wanes: The slow moon climbs:
The deep, moans round with many voices.
Come, my friends, 'tis not too late to seek a newer world.
We are not now that strength which in old days
moved earth and heaven; that which we are, we are;
one equal temper of heroic hearts,
made weak by time and fate,
but strong in will to survive,
to seek, to find, and not to yield."

—Alfred, Lord Tennyson
Ulysses

ACKNOWLEDGMENTS

All memoirs are, to some degree, a catharsis for their author, and this book is no exception. In the process of writing (and rewriting and rewriting), I had a wonderful opportunity to see more clearly what happened and to understand why events unfolded the way they did. This was a great gift to me. But, if I were the only person who benefits, this book would have no meaning. In recounting my experiences, I hope my family, friends, colleagues, and those whom I haven't met, find ideas, emotions, or situations that they identify in their own lives.

Editors exist to make authors look good and I'm extremely grateful to Kitty O'Callaghan for smoothing out my stubborn cowlicks of circular reasoning, trimming rambling sentences, and wiping away any extra commas so I might look a bit more presentable to the public. That Kitty is also my daughter makes my appreciation for her efforts even more profound. I acknowledge and appreciate her literary expertise, and her willingness to see me not only as a father but also as a doctor, and as a writer.

I want to say thank you to Marcia Lorenzen, who came out of retirement as a special favor to me, to copy-edit the manuscript. I'll never use the word "that" again without thinking twice and remembering her in the process. Special thanks go to my graphic designer, Camin Potts, of Graphic Liaisons, LLC, for her elegant cover design, photo placements, and chapter organization, pulling everything together beautifully and professionally.

Finally, I'd like to say thank you to my dedicated wife, Mary. Without her loving support of my endeavors—from the day we met until now—I would not have such a *Heartfelt Journey* to retell.

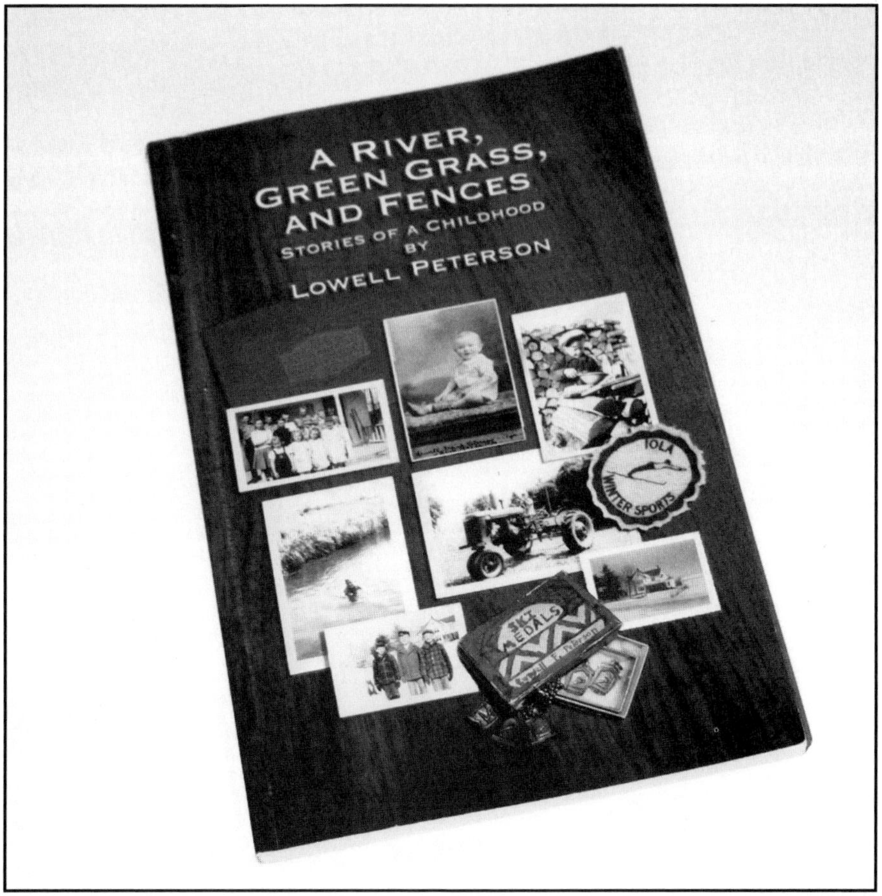

A River, Green Grass, and Fences **Lowell Peterson**

Influenced throughout my childhood by the events of WWII and the early years of the Cold War, my first collections of childhood memoirs take place in the tiny, one-street town of Sheridan, Wisconsin and later on a farm, set in the rolling, glacier-carved hills near Scandinavia, Wisconsin. My childhood world was small—ten miles in any direction covered it. I attended a one-room schoolhouse for eight years and often was the only student in my grade; high school with a total of fifty students followed.

I have never forgotten, nor will I, my idyllic, charmed childhood and my childhood friends. The old haunts we traversed and the fun we had, remain dear to my heart. Enjoy these childhood experiences with me, in a time before TV, video games, computers and the internet, in *A River, Green Grass and Fences*.

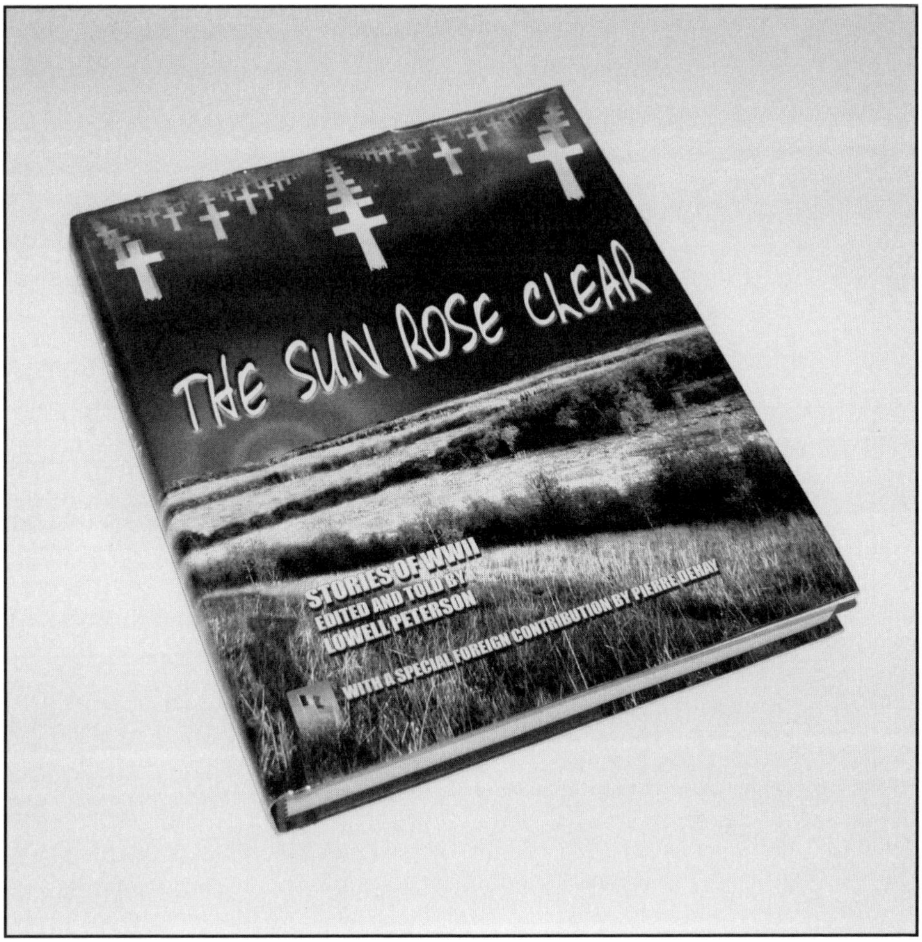

The Sun Rose Clear **Lowell Peterson**

The stories in this book explore an expansive picture of World War II, but more importantly, show the human side of the war through the eyes of men and women who experienced World War II firsthand. *The Sun Rose Clear* is a collection of stories as told to me by my patients. As I accumulated their stories, I felt a sense of urgency to capture as much as I could before their experiences could not be told again. Written and told by them, these war stories recreate the tragedy of war so that the reader can relate to, and relive the actual events as they happened.

I experienced WWII on the homefront, during my childhood, which has lead to my lifelong interest in, and study of, this cataclysmic event. WWII left fifty-five million people dead and twelve million as refugees. It was the single most defining event of the twentieth century.

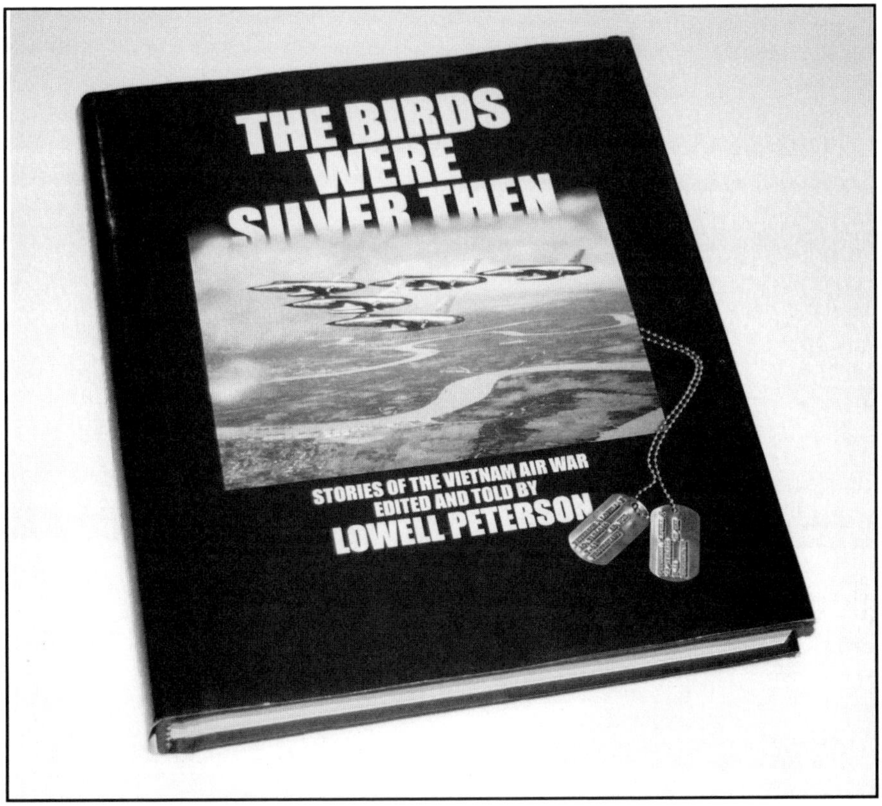

The Birds Were Silver Then **Lowell Peterson**

After writing *The Sun Rose Clear*, I began collecting stories told first-hand by pilots in the U.S. Air Force from 1963-1966, when the majority of the people in the U.S. still felt optimistic about our government's policies. Few understood the increasing danger we faced.

Among the first to engage in combat and to suffer casualties and capture were Navy and Air Force pilots sent on missions into North Vietnam. In *The Birds Were Silver Then* we experience a turning point in the war occurring on July 27, 1965. It was the date of the first attack on the SAM missile sites near Hanoi. What the pilots of the 12th TAC Fighter Squadron and the other F-105 Squadrons endured for this mission illustrates the heroic nature of these brave men, and exemplifies the righteousness of purpose they harbored in their hearts in spite of what they perceived as a horribly misguided strategy and policy. Before that day, the idealism of the pilots remained untarnished.